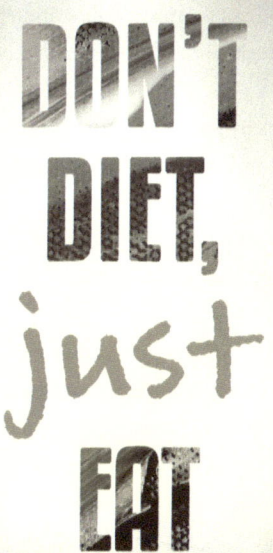

DON'T DIET, just EAT

Trust Your Inner Wisdom, Even When It's Wrong

Katie Nowikow

Don't Diet, Just Eat
Copyright © 2015 by Katie Nowikow

The content of this book is for general instruction only. Each person's physical, emotional, and spiritual condition is unique. The instruction in this book is not intended to replace or interrupt the reader's relationship with a physician or other professional. Please consult your doctor for matters pertaining to your specific health and diet.

To contact the author, visit
www.katiemaehc.com

978-1516950720
1516950720

Printed in the United States of America

paying it forward

To the memory of Peter McWilliams, the man who introduced me to the amazing world of self-help books, whose words in *Life 101* gave me comfort, clarity, and inspiration on my path in life and ultimately inspired me to become a writer and to pay forward help to others the way he did for me.

CONTENTS

Acknowledgements

This book would not be possible without the love and support of some awesome people in life and fellow creative minds.

Mom and Dad–I love you. With love to my family and friends for the support you have given me with every crazy new adventure I take in life.

My amazingly patient and supportive husband who always stands by me, picks me up when I struggle, and lets me be or feel whatever I need to so I can keep moving forward.

To my most amazing, biggest shining star in my life, my son—my biggest accomplishment and joy!

With my deepest gratitude, I want to acknowledge the Institute for Integrative Nutrition, the educators, employees, and founder, Joshua Rosenthal, who put a voice and a reality to the path I was looking for in my life. The experience there was so transformational in my personal and professional life. A sincere thank you for all those involved with the book course program, Lindsey Smith, and all the additional moderators. Without your support, guidance, and united community, I know my book would still be waiting to unfold.

To all those creative minds at Promoting Natural Health, LLC. My editor, Amanda. Your truthfulness was like a breath of fresh air and you challenged me to grow and supported me in the process. I've grown not only as a coach and writer, but as a person. Your support, integrity, brilliance, and honesty are my pillars of strength and confidence in moving me through the writing process.

To Amie - You're a design rockstar! You packaged together this dream of mine into something I can really call my own. Your support, input, and collaboration have been invaluable throughout this process.

To any of the other creative minds with PNH who I may not have had direct contact with–my deepest gratitude and appreciation for all of your hard work and collaboration.

Amber–you are always my sounding board when I feel lost, excited, challenged, unsure or confident, you are always there to stand by me. You helped me to walk the path I needed to most by staying true to myself. Thanks friend, you're awesome and one hell of a coach!

Introduction

You are more than the worries, doubts, imperfections, and little pieces of things on your mind. You are more than your weight, clothing size, skin color, or anything else that holds you back from chasing your dreams and sharing your true self with the world, leaving you frozen in fear in your own web of insecurities.

At the very center of your life is you–this flowing, growing, thinking, learning source of energy. You cannot be placed into a basic box category of this-or-that diet, social clique, or description. It's just not reasonable to expect all of us to fall into one specific way of achieving results by implementing one method for the masses. What *does* work is when people trust themselves to listen to their inner wisdom and take a step in their own way to take care of themselves.

Truth is, the weight loss industry is a money making machine and there's a lot of missing pieces, which is why I'm so thankful for the training I've had–through which I look at you.

Yes, are there different dietary plans and theories in which people not only lose and maintain weight on, but improve their health greatly? Of course. Just as many people heal from dealing with emotional trauma, or changing other pieces of their lives such as career, family situation, living arrangements, or any other number of factors. Some people become healthier when deepening a spiritual practice and change their outlook on life. There's no one way for everyone, there's only the path that you will walk that will be ever unfolding in front of you with each step you take.

You see, the beauty of this entire picture is that you already have exactly what you need to accomplish the goals you have. You don't have to *be* or do anything other than who you are right now in the moment. The solutions, guidance, and answers you find while searching outside of yourself will be yours to see and use as you see fit, as though each resource has information while also holding a mirror reflecting your own internal messages, fears, hopes, and all that lies in between that are hard to see and fully hear without that reflection.

You will begin to hear these messages more clearly when you push past the insecurities, push past the negative voices in your head and mind telling you of all your mistakes or potential mistakes, if you push past all of your fears, and seek out that one calm, patiently waiting voice–the one that says, "Maybe it is just as simple as doing this or that." You will hear your inner wisdom, that voice that will get you through the tough times, will help you determine what step is next– because it is you, your heart, soul, and everything that is you.

When you can stand in alignment with yourself, the healing choices you can make *for you* will open up and resonate with you. What will be good for you today will be different in a week, a month, a year because we are always changing, growing, and exposed to the opportunity to learn.

You are more than your diet, your weight, your outward appearance, and inside insecurities. You are a multi-layered, unique, amazing, imperfect, and worthy person.

Think of your life as a story or a movie. What is so enjoyable about stories and movies, the entire picture? The start, the challenges, the fun times, the big ah-ha's, and the happy ending, right? (Who likes a cliffhanger? I don't! But to each their own.) Is your story going to be all about your dieting woes? No, people want to know *you*.

Live your story and be the rich, full character of yourself, even when that is the unsure, sad, angry, or lost person. It's what you do when you recognize these feelings that matter. I mean, really, would you watch a movie all about a character that is stuck in the diet rut, searching and thinking always about her diet, weight loss, and healthy food? Of course not, and you are more than just this part of your life. Even the big names in the health industry who share their journey usually have some turning point where they, as a person, had to take a leap of faith or tap into their own beliefs to forge ahead, and this is the truth for any journey of growth no matter what it surrounds.

Your life and your days are about much more than food, your size, and the things you don't like. Start living your story and let the layers of what is really ailing you unfold. Because the diet, food, weight loss, it only reaches the surface levels of what is really there. Most of what is put out into the diet industry today is only a surface level solution because there is so much more to what you are experiencing than simply finding the right foods to eat.

In my profession as an integrative nutrition health coach, I get to look beyond food and really look at the individual person, which is my favorite part of my work and it is the key element in helping people to make positive changes for their overall health, not just weight or food choices.

We'll walk through different ways to begin getting in touch with yourself and delving into your many layers so you can find more than one way to engage in self-care and begin taking steps to love yourself and your life. We will look at the ability to hear your inner wisdom by letting yourself off the hook, redefining success, stopping the judgment cycle, and living your story–the good and the bad.

Yes, this is a book with some nutrition information–basic stuff to get you going, to help you support yourself with healthy foods. Yes, there is a lot about emotions, feelings, and facing a variety of challenges, but also walking into opportunities, growing, and learning.

With each step, you can figure out what you need, what is next, and what is for you. Step into the story of your life, start thinking of it in a much bigger picture, bigger than today or the struggles you've had.

You are much more than these experiences in life–we all are. You are enough right now.

one

Don't Diet, Just Eat

Not only should you be living your story, but I want to put the fun and excitement back into your feelings around food. We should be able to enjoy all aspects of food–visual, scent, and taste. It's not instantly bad food just because of what the food item is if the context in which you're having a piece of birthday cake is a joyous experience.

One day, while grocery shopping with my man candy, and walking through the bakery aisles ogling all the treats, my husband asked me, "Why do you torture yourself like that?" He couldn't understand, since I'd gone gluten-free and couldn't eat any of these foods anymore, why I wanted to look at all of it.

To which I replied, with a big smile, "Well, I guess I'm gluten for punishment!" I was so proud. I knew my mom would be proud at that head shaker! I loved baked goods, and part of that love is just looking at all the pretty decorated globs of icing and colors and seeing the different flavor combos. Most of the time, I don't want to eat all of what I see because I know that my icing is better.

We have become so conditioned to look at foods as bad or good, and healthy is only attained by a certain way. But it should be something to enjoy, to fully experience, not loathe or dread. Health food doesn't have to be bland and boring and uneventful. Part of how we got here with food is the four letter word. D-I-E-T. The twisty, toxic relationship of good versus evil! You know the one. It goes like this.

Monday, I'm starting my diet. New Year, new diet. New season to feel good in your clothes. All different common times to start your diet. New day, week, or month. The sales are all the same—start here, finish there, this is what you are promised, and if you can hack it, this is what you will get.

Most of us always find our ears perking up at the latest and greatest advertisement offering your perfect body on a silver platter with just a few "simple" secret steps in exchange for a lump of cash. The weight loss industry appeals to the masses with one message: we have the answers you need to get and stay thin. The underlying message is: if you can do it. The same marketing is dressed differently for each changing season be it New Year resolutions or getting ready for swimsuit season.

One-size-fits-all plans and products are being pushed as though it really should be just that simple. Want to lose weight? Well, I'll tell you what to eat, when and how, and it'll work for you and everyone you know, as though everyone who wants to lose weight is just one big problem to which there is one simple solution. But nowhere in the fine print does it address what happens when said plans don't work for the individual other than, "What did you do wrong?"

We are at an unhealthy crossroads with food in our culture. Cheap, processed, salty, sugary, fatty, and nutritionally empty foods are everywhere. Office parties, social events, gas stations, drug stores, just about any retailer has candy and soft drinks available at the checkout line. This doesn't even include restaurants, commercial advertisements, and visual cues for food that we see, smell, or hear about.

Having grown up eating processed foods, it is common for most of us to develop a taste palette accustomed to these types of empty calorie foods. This interferes with the tastes of healthy foods, something that takes time to acquire an appreciation for different flavors, which is not a luxury provided in most dieting plans.

To combat the never ending supply of empty calorie foods is the never ending newest, latest, and greatest product, plan, or service to lose weight, get in shape, and look great! But, it all rests on you! If you can't follow this plan to a T, you'll fail and it'll be all your fault and you won't ever get healthy. So you try this plan or that plan and when you can't hack it, well, it is your failure and it weighs you down. So the dieting industry comes out on top smelling like roses because it worked for *these* people—what's wrong with you?

Dieting, as in the act of going on a diet, regardless of *what* plan it may be, often requires drastic measures that are not practical. I think of dieting in the following context. It is an unforgiving process leaving little to no room for imperfection, mistakes, or normal human error, and requires extreme tactics of doing it all at once to force quick results and then hope those results will provide continued motivation to keep going.

Dieting requires starting at the finish line with the routine, but not with the results. It's like trying to run your first 5K at the lowest time of the best runner instead of running at your own pace. You know how it goes. You pick your start date and then are encouraged to buy into all the recommended foods, products, supplements, whatever, and you start full force doing each meal differently and forcing an exercise routine, both of which may or may not fit your needs.

These intense measures are how we get drastic results, right? Sure, sometimes, for a little bit, maybe. The all-or-nothing traditional approach consists of a drastic overhaul happening in a short period of time. The idea being if you just rip the bandage off, maybe you'll finally give up fast food, soda, or sugar for good. Maybe if I make it twenty, thirty, or ninety days with non-processed foods, I'll suddenly love vegetables. Maybe. Or maybe you'll quit after ten days, drive your loved ones up a wall with your stunning personality during this "challenge," and down a box of Krispy Kreme on your way to Taco Bell singing "Free Falling" at the top of your lungs.

Extreme measures allow no room for error and also promote deprivation! Just say no! I hear the advertisements for a variety of supplements on the radio for appetite suppression and it kills me every time. You're hungry for nutritionally empty foods because that's what your mind is translating from your physical hunger, so here, we'll just nix that instinctual desire to eat altogether, instead of say, just having a healthy snack.

Here are a few of the other tried and true methods used in weight loss that often become a part of the problem instead of the solution. An oldie and an assumed goodie—calorie tracking or food journaling. The goodie side—these are great tools to gather data and establish a baseline of your habits, understand where your calories are coming from, and to get a feel for what you're doing or eating, or what's triggering certain habits.

Calorie tracking is great for those numbers people, or for those who like to know how things work, this can be a very informational process and may work for some in that respect. Food journaling can be great when used to identify the emotional relationship between food and eating habits. Both can provide a sense of accountability or accomplishment when making progress toward change or getting a handle on the habits surrounding poor food choices. I'm not at all saying it should never be used or isn't helpful. I am saying that forcing it isn't going to guarantee results, nor does this actually provide positive motivation for *everyone*.

Yet somehow, it is seen as vital to being successful. I promise you that you can still make healthy changes, lose weight, and improve your eating habits without using these tools. To be healthy doesn't mean you log your calories or track each meal. For me, personally, I'm not a fan of this past the point of gathering some baseline information or awareness, and I'll encourage a person to use this tool if and when it works to create positive motivation through insight into their own struggles and ways to overcome these struggles.

I have never tracked my calories. Never. Not once. Even when I was trying to skip fast food and lose a little weight to fit into my favorite pair of jeans, I still never tracked my calories. I always thought it was complicated to determine how many calories to burn and how many I needed to take in on a daily basis. To be quite honest, when I was eating bad food, I knew I was eating bad food and it was because it was greasy and could clog my arteries or make me sick in other ways. Calories were never really on my radar. I mean, most of us know the drive-thru meal isn't very good for us? Right.

This is why you feel bad and guilty when you finish the double cheeseburger meal with fries and a trough of soda. You know you aren't doing well for yourself with your food choices. I didn't need yet another reinforcement telling me I was doing badly by tracking my calories or fat intake. It didn't motivate me. It scared the crap out of me and made me feel anxious and uncomfortable, and it reinforced the feelings that put me in the drive-thru in the first place.

Constantly micromanaging your food can also become a bit tedious and consuming, and often leads to more stress and rigidity. It makes it more about the foods than about you, and it's about you first. Healthy living isn't about being rigid or uptight, or always perfect and on task. It's about taking care of yourself, and believe it or not, self-care isn't supposed to be challenging and no fun.

Weight loss driven dieting impacts you personally, in your social life, financially, well, basically in every capacity of your life. Ever go to work on the office birthday cake day when starting your diet? Oh ya. What about your friend's party or the holiday get together? All awful times to be on a diet. This is when most of us fall off the wagon, and for some, this leads to another bender of many days full of guilt and shame for doing bad once, so what's the point in trying again? Been there, done that.

Dieting is not automatically synonymous with health as there are many plans that are not at all healthy but you can lose weight on, and this includes the mental or emotional health during the process of dieting. Much of the overly advertised dieting methods are geared for quick results around weight loss only, and with most people being pressed for time, short on cash, and being pulled in a million directions, the desire to feel good about ourselves, our bodies, and have more energy is strong. And we. Want. It. Yesterday. Of course, that means to have it now, that means I have to do it all right now. I have to be good. Start my diet on Monday with no looking back.

Marketing feeds this mentality even more so with smoke and mirrors advertising. Vague details eluding to weight loss results that last, leaving it all on you to do the work required to obtain said results.

Most importantly, you are left out of the equation when it comes to dieting, both on a physical and personal level.

With many of us consuming the standard American diet high in processed, sugary, salty, fatty foods, and not a lot of nutritionally dense foods, we now have a new host of health issues including, but not limited to, our ever expanding waste lines. In turn, we have quite the buzz around different types of foods, ways of eating, and everyone wants to be king of the mountain with the *right* answer.

If I follow suit with this pattern, it would be easy for me to hammer down some plan mirroring the personal experience I have had with food over the years and to simply tell you to do what I do, because it worked for me. I have tried this approach, but now, anytime someone asks me for an eating plan or a set program to abide by, I get uncomfortable and feel the lack of my ability to provide such a plan or program. Because a set plan will not be nearly as valuable as taking the time to work with you as an individual. I want to help you find your own way.

I am not going to write yet another book on nutrition when there are already a TON of other resources available. I will, however, provide you with basic nutrition information to help you shop for healthy foods and have healthier meals. I could get into a lot of fancy words like macronutrients or yin and yang food qualities, but most of us live a crazy, busy, demanding life, and it doesn't have to be so complicated. We need to step back to food basics and just get simple with things. Everything is so intense these days. Do I have enough super foods, am I eating the right kind of peanut butter, do I buy low-fat or low-sodium or kosher? Labels, advertisements, and buzz words further complicate this problem.

I will give you the tools to implement basic, small changes in your daily life that will enable learning, personal growth, and confidence in taking care of yourself. With these tools and techniques, you will be able to let go of past attempts that weigh you down with feelings of frustration and failure. You will be able to pick out a diet plan better suited for your needs and lifestyle. You will be able to use the one variable everyone is overlooking, yourself. That is the strongest asset you have available to yourself.

This book is part of the self-health movement. We cannot continue to compartmentalize ourselves, seeking single solutions for the masses to resolve a multitude of complex and individualized problems. To simplify a problem and find somewhere to get started, I love breaking it down Barney style. That's pretty much my M.O.

To continually break things up, compartmentalize, and define everything into a neat little box or category is missing the point, and leaving more important pieces out of the picture. Instead, let's begin to understand that our relationship with food, movement, and overall physical, mental, and emotional health is somehow separated from our level of satisfaction in life, from our overall sense of happiness. This will continue to deliver the same temporary or empty results. All of these parts of ourselves and our lives are intertwined into a beautiful combination of our being.

Even our bodies are treated as individual parts though the entire system functions together. We act as though our tailbone isn't connected to our hip bone. (Yay, side effects of parenthood!)

One of the most helpful aspects of working with a coach is having the chance to speak up and have a safe place to express your feelings—be it feelings of failure or feelings of doubt or feelings of what you want to do versus what you *should* do. After having a safe place to speak to someone, be heard, validated, and encouraged to walk your own path, most people find they are able to see positive results.

It's like getting permission, and though I'm not actually giving anyone permission, the validation and the discussion provides the same feeling of getting the permission to go ahead with whatever someone may be thinking about doing.

Coaches, I and others, provide you a safe space to be heard so your inner wisdom can come through. Sometimes we just need to hear from someone else, "Yes, that is okay, go with it."

You will get results by doing things your own way. Let's start by embracing the one overlooked variable in the diet and weight loss saga–*you*. Everyone is different and everyone will have their own stories, needs, struggles, and ways of making changes. Our gender, age, medical history, ethnicity, blood type, upbringing, etc. all contribute to how our bodies are going to use and respond to food. Not to mention, any emotional or life experiences you have tied to food create a truly individual fingerprint of characteristics specific to you and your way of life with food.

Just keep in mind, according to the dictionary, a diet simply means "one's usual food," or "special food taken as health."

Can diets be helpful for you when they fit the definition of "special food taken as health?" You bet! This means you will get help and results in healing and reaching your goals with weight or health. Diet also means what you're eating or not eating. And last but not least, the weight loss industry and the gimmick diets in today's industry are failing us, but the picture doesn't stop there. Much more is left to be considered.

– two –

Just Tell Me What to Eat

"Just tell me what to eat!" hands up in the air, surrendering to frustration. This is what I've felt like and have heard a lot. There's so much ever changing information on nutrition that it can be downright exhausting to figure out what to do, if it's right or right just for today, and where to start.

So we are going to get this one knocked out right now– the, "What should I eat?" There is much more information to cover, but this is the yearning question I get all of the time. Yet, most of us already know the answer because we all usually know most of, maybe not all, but most of the foods that we eat when they are unhealthy foods, right?

Here is the simple starting point for learning more about nutrition. When buying packaged food items, read the ingredient label—not the marketing on the front, not the nutrition panel with your calculator in hand to determine what equals what. Look at the ingredient panel to see *what is in your food*.

Next, go back to basics. If you were to think of meals from one hundred years ago, what would the food consist of? I don't mean specifics of each individual type of vegetable or fruit or what kind of meat, but it'd likely consist of *real food*. Preservatives were salt, sugar, or fat and in much lesser amounts.

Start first with home cooked meals, even if it's pizza or burgers and fries. You can prepare the food in healthier ways than a restaurant, you can make your portions smaller, and ultimately, it'll be a much healthier meal.

Do two things. Pick your biggest food vice and the foods you like the least. For me, that was sugar and vegetables. Focus on adding more vegetables to your meals–and don't fret about how they are cooked. True story about two food items and how I acquired a taste for them. Broccoli and strawberries. I really didn't like broccoli unless I ordered it from a restaurant and it was cooked, well, usually with butter and a little cheese on top. But I was awful at making it myself, always overcooked it. One of my regular lunch spots during work had great burgers, so I'd get a cheeseburger and broccoli. The broccoli somehow magically absorbed the taste of the burger and was just the right texture. While it's still not the top of my favorite vegetable list, I do like broccoli and can now eat it without being hamburger flavored.

Same thing with strawberries. Yes, there was actually a time when I didn't like something as sweet and tasty as a strawberry. But when you grow up eating sugary desserts and fast food, it's easy to see how that might happen.

I love chocolate and I'd get a jar of hot fudge topping for ice cream and I'd have a huge bowl of strawberries with a sizeable dollop of chocolate sauce to dip then in. It was a favorite treat and I figured this was a compromise to have fruit with my chocolate. Another one I liked was grapes and cool whip. One day, while putting my groceries away and feeling rather hungry, I was snacking on random things when it occurred to me, "Yes, you did just eat a strawberry without chocolate sauce, and liked it." It didn't take long before I'd have them without the chocolate sauce or much less of it.

So don't get hung up on not using dressing, sauce, butter, cheese, salt or pepper, or chocolate to eat healthy foods. Season it, flavor it, dunk it, drown it, and just eat it. Some way or another, eat it. (Okay, well, don't batter it, deep fry it, and then dunk it in ketchup. That wouldn't really work.) Focus on getting the nutrition into your body, and remember, you are learning to acquire a taste for these foods.

Start small by adding healthy foods to your regular meals—frozen, fresh, or canned, just eat them. Get what you can afford, what you can cook, and what you will eat. It is still better than not having anything at all. Start small and make big changes. Your body will send you signals saying, "Hey, I want more of that stuff."

It's not the same way you crave pizza or doughnuts with enough force to take out a small army to get your treat. It's more of a natural desire to just eat, and you'll begin to choose the healthy meal over the pizza because you'll know how crappy the pizza will make you feel and it won't be worth it, whereas the healthy meal will taste good and you won't feel like crap afterward, nor will you have the guilt storm going on in your mind. And with the acquired taste, the healthier meals will become more appealing. I'm not yankin' your chain on this one. Do you know I actually get excited to go to some restaurants and get appetizers that are all vegetables? It's true. And not deep fried into unrecognizable vegetable oblivion either.

It's natural to expect that after so long of eating different kinds of flavors you may not just like other types. If you try a certain fruit or vegetable a few times and don't seem to like it when you cook, order it when you dine out and try it that way. If you still don't like it, move on to the next vegetable to try.

I'm going to tell you a little something that'll save you a lot of time and energy. The quality dietary theory plans are very much alike, and they all have a common ground to stand on that usually starts with exploring basic advice about these things:

- Cutting out sugar-in foods and drinks
- Eliminating processed foods
- Increasing water intake
- High intake of plant foods—fruits, vegetables, grains, legumes, nuts and seeds (any combination of, or some and not others)

That's it. The rest—how you cook it, whether it is organic or not, and the specific foods you eat or don't eat—all vary with each plan, as they should.

The other elements of different dietary theories consist of a few different things. First, what is it for?

- Based on a region of the world and their natural and indigenous foods
- Based on cultures of people, but on the time they existed rather than where they existed
- Inclusive of bigger life practices beyond food–meditation, exercise, spiritual practices
- Personal or ethically based

For instance, the Ayurvedic Diet is much more than a diet of what foods to eat and not eat. Based out of India, this is an approach for not only the body, but for the mind to create balance within and with nature. Five doshas represent the different elements of nature—fire, air, water, and earth. It is believed, in Ayurveda, that being out of alignment with oneself and nature results in disease.

The five doshas, or elements, are used to describe different body types, physical characteristics, and personalities, with most of us having multiple doshas, one primary and the rest secondary. The different body types give an outline of what types of food to incorporate, and unlike other dietary plans where one is following a set list of foods, this modality incorporates six different tastes: Sour, sweet, salty, strong, bitter, and acidic. Each of these different tastes has its own healing properties most effective in application by eating a combination.

Additionally, practicing meditation, yoga, breathing exercises, doing cleanses, and/or use of herbal oils are also part of this method.

Within this one theory, the individual is recognized and there is much more to consider than simply which super food to eat and what to avoid as it is all about the entire picture of having one's life in balance. Which body type you are determines which types of foods you should eat, what types of activities you should do, and what element you are.

In figuring out if you want to follow a plan and which one to choose from, it is helpful to look at these different factors of a theory when going down this road. It also will show the depth, credibility, and practicality of these plans or theories for you.

A busy individual with work and family demands may not have the time to jump into an Ayurvedic way of living.

As with most things, there is always controversy surrounding which plan is the best or the *right* one to follow, and we'll look into this more in depth when reviewing the theory of bio-individuality, but for now, let's just get back to answering the basic question of, "What should I eat?"

Eat food, real food. Read your ingredients. Cook more at home when you can. Most of us know when we're eating unhealthy food items because we feel bad about it. That guilt is hanging around there just waiting to jump on the attack once the meal is finished, or sometimes before you've left the drive-thru.

Here are some simple questions you can ask yourself when thinking of what to eat:

- Does it come from a plant, animal, or a factory?
- Is it the type of food that makes me want to eat and eat and eat, and then have ice cream?
- Do I know I'll feel like crap after having this meal?

Now for more nutrition information, I'm not going to rewrite perfection so I'll refer you to a great book by Michael Pollan called *Food Rules: An Eater's Manual.* This book is invaluable, easy to read, easy to understand, and well, perfect.

Sometimes it's not even just about *what* you're eating, it is about where what you are eating comes from. Is it at home, or from the drive-thru? At a restaurant, from the gas station, or grocery store salad bar? Is it coming out of packages, or is any of it fresh produce or fresh foods?

Or it may be looking at *when* you are eating and how often. Are you over eating or eating just enough food? Are you eating late at night and skipping meals during the day time?

You see, there are many questions to consider when thinking about our habits with food and how to implement changes. The most important question, though, is not the what, when, or how much. No. The most important question is *why* am I eating foods I know are not good for me, and *why* do I not want to eat the foods that are good for me? That, my friend, is where the answers lie.

– three –

Primary Foods

Just as we are with food, we are in complicated times with our daily lives and lifestyle. People are overworked, underpaid, misconnected, multi-tasking, on information overload, and just plain worn out. Don't get me wrong, it ain't all bad, but there definitely seem to be some things working against us, right?

Primary foods encompass the most basic concepts of self-care by aligning your personal needs in the areas of career, relationships, physical activity, and spirituality as being vital components to your overall health and wellbeing. Taking care of yourself allows you to be better suited and energized to care for others, be it your immediate family and friends or bigger communities in your life. Though we hear it or say it to ourselves repeatedly, it is often much more difficult to apply in our lives. Secondary foods go in your face – FOOD!

Today, in Western culture, many of us have huge deficiencies in these areas of our lives. We're blinded by responsibility, by social and peer pressure, fear of failure or success, or feelings of guilt for taking time to do what you *want* to do, or feeling selfish for wanting too much out of life for yourself.

These areas suffer with sentiments similar to, "Nothing's perfect and I live in the *real world*," or, "You can't be too picky, sometimes you just have to suck it up," or, "It must be nice to have it so easy/be so lucky/know the right people."

All of these say the same underlying thing: I don't believe good things are possible for me. When you think others are lucky and somehow better or more deserving of something than you are, it begins to create this unattainable edge to their life that you cannot, and will not, have. Like luck is something you are born with or without.

Maybe we need to accept the possibility of having good things as being normal rather than expecting the mundane. But does anyone really set out to engage in mundane friendships or careers? I don't think so. At some point, along the line of being hurt, feeling insecure, failing, and being taught how to be responsible in the name of safety, we lose sight of why it is important, normal, and healthy to seek out the parts of ourselves that shine, and to give them the opportunity to shine in all capacities of our lives.

But what if I don't have anything to offer? I'm not special, or creative, or different. I'm just an average person. To which I say, "Share your brownies!"

A profound lecture I once heard discussed this notion of holding back and not giving ourselves, thoughts, and ideas to others as similar to having a plate full of brownies at a party and hogging them in the corner and not sharing. Brilliant! Though I'd totally hide the brownies for myself! (Bonus to being the weird healthy one in my family is that now my brownies usually have some foreign, obscurely hidden healthy ingredient so my family always hesitates to eat them…ha! More chocolate for me!)

When you are happy and fulfilled, you have that much more to offer others. I can tell you now in my life, being healthier mentally and physically, I can focus on bigger problems. I can give back more to others in my community and am more engaged in finding ways to make tomorrow a better day. But when I was bogged down with insecurities, feeling like crap, and loathing going to work each day, I didn't have any spare energy or willpower left to give to anyone besides Ben & Jerry. Now, however, I want to share my brownies.

Don't underestimate your brownie and what it has to offer because you never know how much joy, comfort, hope, entertainment, or inspiration you provide to another person by doing what you do, by just being you. But you can't be the best version of yourself without actually providing yourself with the same care and attention you'd give to anyone else.

Ask yourself this: Does it really make sense to spend all of your time and energy in areas of your life just because you *have to* without there also being a bigger driver or win at stake? I'm all for responsibility. I've been there, done that. That doesn't mean you can't be working toward a place where *have to* and *want to* become one in the same.

Deficiencies in primary foods trigger secondary food choices, and poor secondary food choices compound the stress associated with primary foods since they provide instant temporary relief, comfort, or entertainment. Wouldn't it be a nice break to focus your energy somewhere else instead of just on your diet and exercise?

Well, you can, because when there is a deficiency in a primary food area, it can carry over into other areas of your life and, as I mentioned, affect your food choices. When I was completely lost without an idea of what to do with my professional life and working in a job in which I wasn't making enough money nor feeling as though my forty hours a week were spent enriching my life, but more like a never ending cycle of pushing myself to just make it through one more day, this spilled into my personal life. I'd spend nights on the couch dreading the next day of work, crying from feeling lost without a clear direction, and having to waste yet another day of my life doing empty work. This affected my desire to enjoy many things including engaging in self-care activities such as cooking healthy meals or exercising. The stress was physically and mentally exhausting.

The easiest part of primary foods is seeing the problem. The hard part is figuring out the solution to these problems and not getting stuck in it, but moving through it toward the light at the end of the tunnel.

Health is not a possession or a final place. It is a way of living that encompasses all things beyond our plate or weight. It encompasses the choices you make, the way you live your life, your feelings of purpose. Each of these areas directly shape the others because you are at the center of it all, and you bring to each different area of your life the feelings, happiness, and purpose of yourself.

Each area of primary foods represents how your life's energy is being spent and replenished. If your career is suffering, your energy is going to be spent unevenly by trying to manage surviving your career and its challenges. When you're engaging in unfulfilling or toxic relationships, your energy is going to be expended quickly and exhaustively in dealing with these relationships. The list goes on and on in each area of your life. The most damaging reality of it being that your energy is taken, used, or exhausted *without* being positively replaced or charged to give you the boost of happiness and excitement you would be experiencing in different circumstances.

At the root of all these potential primary food deficiencies are the emotions, beliefs, and abilities you feel you have that can create or lead to imbalances and deficiencies in one or multiple areas of your life. It's the center of you, what you feel, perceive, and create. This is how and where change can take shape and place.

When dealing with primary food challenges, you are not a whole person, you are going to be experiencing your life with missing pieces. It is part of the experience of life to have a deficiency, imbalance, or missing piece, but it's what you do to create balance and fulfill the deficiency that counts as well as what you learn along the way.

Let me elaborate here and explain what I mean each of these things to represent:

Imbalance: Super happy with your relationship, super happy with a workout routine, really unhappy with finances or work. An imbalance left stagnant or unresolved for too long will develop into a deficiency.

Deficiency: One or more primary foods are completely draining and it's impacting the amount of joy and pleasure you're able to experience in other parts of your life.

Missing pieces: These are a little more enigmatic in that you may know something, but you don't even know it yet because you are first, naturally focusing on the clearly defined imbalances or deficiencies, but in time, it'll surface and you'll wonder, "How did I ever miss this?"

No matter what you are dealing with, when you experience any or all of these, there are many ways to provide temporary and quick distractions and indulgences, be it shopping, eating, gambling, sleeping, or what have you, there are many ways to compensate in an empty fashion. Food, specifically fast food and sugar, was my vice.

It wasn't long ago I had a freezer with six cartons of ice cream taking up residence. I'm not kidding, six cartons. Today, I'm in a much better place, yet I still do not feel I've arrived at "health." I do believe I follow a healthy lifestyle, which means I am open to learning, challenging my comfort zone, and trying to continue to find and consume nourishing foods. It is much more than a temporary feeling of arrival. It means I get to continually "arrive" at different destinations—way cool!

I have managed to let go of a lot of choices and ways of life that were no longer serving me by changing my life, finding a line of work I truly felt called to do, finding a partner to build a life and family with, finding support with wellness practitioners (who rock!), and by also paying more attention to how food affects my mind and body. At the center of all of these actions was me, myself, and I. I was taking care of myself.

Ultimately, I did not make lifestyle changes. I changed my

life by working through each deficiency and imbalance. In time, the missing pieces began to pop up and the growth taking place has been much more than finding "the right diet."

As I began to recognize I was the only one in my way of improving my professional path, and that I was also the one who had all the ability to do something about it, I began slowly but surely making changes. I first found my calling by discovering the Institute for Integrative Nutrition. I eventually got a better paying job, though it was still not fulfilling, it did alleviate some of the financial stress I'd been feeling.

With each step I made, I grew more as an individual, and eventually, one little change at a time, this led me away from needing food to be my excitement in life. It led me away from needing to waste money on stuff that'd only provide temporary happiness. I remember the first time I turned down McDonalds French fries without even a second thought. A co-worker of mine had gotten an extra bag of fries by mistake or something. She was walking around offering some fries to people and asked me, and without hesitation, I was like, "Oh, I'm good thanks." To clarify, I grew up on chicken McNuggets and French fries from McDonalds, seriously, and French fries are still one of my favorite foods.

A couple minutes after that happened, I thought to myself, "Wait a minute. What just happened? Did I actually turn down French fries because I really don't *want* them?" It was like a moment from the Twilight Zone or something. I had to do a silent happy dance in my cubicle because I felt so proud.

Primary foods suffer for many reasons. It may be the messages we were taught while growing up about these different areas in life. It may be the fears we carry or because we feel inadequate, selfish, or irresponsible to pursue the things we most want out of life. It may feel selfish of you to think YOU can have a career you enjoy and get paid for it. You may feel as though your relationship is normal even though it brings you more stress than joy, but that's how everyone has it, right?

Oh, yes, settling is what so many of us do best. Settling for the responsible path, or the safe and sure way of life. I tried settling many times in my life, mostly because I wasn't fired up about the work it'd take to achieve big goals. Also because I didn't know what the heck to do with myself or my life. I kept looking for something easy, something to pay my bills, make me happy, no risk, no fluff, just easy.

I never used to get that drive they show in movies and TV when someone is working hard to reach a goal. What I didn't know, because I hadn't experienced it yet, was the feeling of excitement when finding something I really believed in and having that fire lit within.

You see, when you find your purpose, passion, calling, or truth, the work becomes almost commonplace because it feels so rewarding to engage in this activity that you just run with it. Yes, you still have challenges, fears, and demons to overcome, but they get run over with the force of a Black Friday shopper chasing the latest deal. They don't stand a chance when faced with passion, hope, and the fulfillment of a true calling.

Figure out where your primary food deficiencies are, and use this other area of getting well to help you overall to feel better about yourself. This will work because there is no better way to invest in yourself than to make sure your life is looking the way you want it to. Remember, primary food deficiencies can be the driving force to the drive-thru window or back to the cookie jar. If you eliminate the triggers by improving your life, cake just is cake, not a huge deal.

Once upon a time, reading something like this, I'd be thinking to myself, "There aren't enough hours in the day to do *what I want* to do. I'm so tired and done when I'm home from work, how will I ever find a new job?"

Wrong. You have time each day, but how you are spending your time is the question. Yes, you have things you *have* to do. That's just life. And in even a few minutes a day you can contribute to big results and get one step closer to improving an imbalance or deficiency in primary foods.

But who says what you have to do cannot lead to, or eventually become synonymous with what you *enjoy*. When you are spending more of your time engaging in a life you enjoy, you will be more energized from your day instead of drained by it. Suddenly, the little acts of self-care that seem so daunting now, won't seem to be such a big deal.

I have a lot of residual angst from working a long time without fulfilling my true calling, and I know how much this can impact overall health, happiness, and opportunity for growth and learning. I also hear it all of the time from a lot of people, be it professionally or personally. Whether it's the career or relationships, any deficiency in your primary foods and you're going to feel the strain of it in your life.

Each area will be a unique process of learning and unfolding opportunities. Start making improvements in the most obvious area because there is likely one overshadowing the others, screaming for attention. With each step toward improving these areas, you'll come across opportunities for change and improvement you may not have even realized.

The cool thing about the process of focusing on your primary foods is that, in time, you will begin to piece it all together in your own way. You start with the area that needs the most attention and you work from there. Listening to your inner wisdom, learning how to let your emotions be of use to you, not hiding or feeling ashamed will get you in touch with your inner wisdom.

Alternately, when you have a better sense of yourself in all of these major life areas, you will be better able to face challenges, to chase your dreams, and to find other means to feel fulfilled beyond your weight, food choices, and clothing size. Wouldn't it be nice to have a break from overanalyzing food choices and calorie counting? Well, you can.

Enriching these areas of your life will bring you other joy that will not only make food just seem like food, it will shape your confidence and sharpen your purpose. All of these areas in your life will either enhance your ability to fulfill your purpose or detract from it.

Sometimes it is the little things in primary foods that are overlooked the most, the little things we get so excited about as kids and as adults but just don't do because we "shouldn't," like staying up too late or playing dress up, eating dessert first or having a snack while cooking, or leaving the dishes sit and reading a book instead.

"You mean, I can do that?" Yes. You can. You should. Is the world going to fall apart when you put off your laundry or dishes for a few hours or a day? Are you going to really regret wearing a flashy new outfit even if it puts you outside your comfort zone?

If it's something bigger like taking a risk on a career pursuit or a chance with love or moving to a new place, you may be hesitant, but what if you never try and are always left wondering? What if you pursue a new career path and you don't make money? Is it really what's going to matter most to you one day when you're thinking back on all the things you didn't do?

Sure, there are poor financial decisions, I'm not saying hit the slots and throw it all away on random and poorly calculated chance, nor do I mean risking yourself or others overall welfare by making snap decisions without considering its impact on all involved.

I am saying to really invest in yourself, find something that'll challenge you to work hard but gives you endless passion! It'll be your own success, your own adventure. This can be confused with being spontaneous, throwing caution to the wind. It's as though once we get a little pep in our step to go after what we want it's like, "Heck with it, I'm all in baby," and the journey begins!

NO, I mean really figure out what you want, improve it, one

at a time, because your dreams shouldn't be about careless or reckless decisions. In some instances, that'll only set you up for failure that much more because you'll put yourself in a more desperate situation. Going for the things that make you tick take work, and yes, there is risk or chance involved, but that risk is often simply putting yourself out there, being open to all of the experiences you may have while chasing your dreams.

At the end of the day, feeding yourself primary foods is another way of saying, "It's all about *me*."

four

You Are Emotional—and That's Okay

Emotions are a part of our natural being and they signal the need for change. They are the guiding force *through* changes on a mental and physical basis as we experience all life has to offer. The engagement of emotional expression may not change the situation you are in, but *you* change before, during, and after your emotional energy response. By doing so, your mentality, reaction, and resilience through emotional turmoil and the challenges life inevitably will throw at us will allow you to adapt, cope, and survive.

When you're not in touch with your emotions, you don't allow your emotions to be expressed around something that bothers you, say for instance, like hating your job. A lot of people aren't happy in their profession, yet tell themselves there are reasons to just deal with it. "People have it much worse than you, you are taking things for granted," or, "those dream jobs don't exist, you can't make money doing something you like."

We find a lot of reasons to justify shutting down and to not engage in what our emotional response is trying to tell us. It's not just letting sadness or anger out by only acknowledging you're not happy at work and venting about it to others. The next step of engaging in our emotional response is saying,

43

"I'm going to *do* something about it," so we don't get stuck in this constant battle of feeling as though we shouldn't be feeling bad, angry, or sad about anything to begin with, as though the feelings themselves need to be ignored or battled.

Instead say, "Hmm, work really stresses me out and I need to change my working environment and set a goal for something that'll make me happy that I can work toward." It's not the same as quitting your job right away and doing what you love and hoping money will come in.

If we are not engaging in our emotions, which these are the first responders to our levels of satisfaction in primary food areas of life, then deficiencies and imbalances will begin to develop. All the while, we continue to fight or ignore whatever emotional stuff is below the surface affecting our mind-body connection for health and wellbeing. Western medicine, the diet industry, social classifications, and our culture in general compartmentalizes everything as we do. But as easy as it would be to break us all up into different categories, we are all much more complex and interesting.

Our emotional health is very important, but emotions are often dismissed as inconvenient, embarrassing, or out of control or childish. So we are always working on being emotionally appropriate to fit in with social or familial expectations. It's often touted the best approach is a positive mindset.

I look at a positive mindset as working within your capacity, of what you have available to you. A positive mindset is just like positive numbers or negative numbers—you either have something or you don't. Even in moments of anger, you can still work within a positive mindset to look at what is in your capacity to do.

All of this ties together with your health and wellbeing, including weight. Are you emotionally spent from fighting, denying, or limiting your emotions and stuck in the, "I'm unhappy at work/in my relationship/or other primary food area, but there's nothing I can do to change these things, but I can feel better about me if I lose weight?" Instead of looking at it from that angle, we need to look at it as, "I'm not happy in this primary food area. I want do to something to change it, and I can do something to change it. In the meantime, I can deal with today's stress by doing, X, Y Z." Then, work toward changing those deficiencies and imbalances in primary foods, which are triggers for unwanted habits like emotional eating. Work toward fixing the things that your emotions are responding to.

Give yourself the space and freedom to say, "You know what, I'm a human being and I'm going to be emotional. It's going to go up and down and change and be imperfect. I'm going to need to express it sometimes, and it is what it is." Find healthy ways to express your feelings by using that positive mindset to look at it strictly as inventory. "Well, what do I have that I can work with? I know I'm unhappy at my job, I know that I need to make an income, I know that there are things I like to do in a working environment that I could tie into work for more personal satisfaction in my profession. I already have this kind of training, and these are my personal connections I can reach out to." This is what I already know I have, which is a positive mindset.

You can still feel angry, which is just the desire to change.

Let that anger be present until it's not useful anymore by letting it run its course. Then, get energized by focusing on those positive elements of what you do have. This is a way to create the change you are looking for. When you start to create the change you are looking for, you're going to find that happiness will present itself.

Happiness is a creative, productive, growing, and evolving energy. It lets us create and give beyond ourselves. It's doing things, making things happen. If anger is the desire for change, then happiness is what happens when you start getting the change by being productive and making change happen. That's why when people are at a place of feeling happy, they are able to give more to other people because you have more creative energy thriving on the act of change. You are an element of changing, growing, and moving. This will help your mind and body.

Think about emotions in the sense that they are there for us to feel, they are not there to change the situation we are in. Emotions are there to help *us* manage the situation we are in, carry us through it, protect us. I will say, I have fought crying like I fight puking. "No, no, I don't want to cry. It hurts too much! I don't want to throw up, it's so gross!" Even though I know I'm going to feel better after the fact, I fight it. It's because it's unpleasant to puke and it's unpleasant and painful to cry. When we think of crying as being weak or too sensitive, "Don't be a crybaby, suck it up, be tough and grunt," it's actually really damn hard to let these feelings out in times of loss, pain, fear, or guilt. It's really exhausting to recognize the full physical and mental capacity of what you are experiencing to just get it all out.

But when you get through a good cry and you fall asleep, or are finally exhausted and feel like, "I have no tears left to cry," you've changed. Your body has taken all that internal emotional energy and found a way to express it, to physically release all that you're feeling but may not be able to say. And it's changed *you*. Yes, your situation may be the same, but you are different. You are one step closer to looking at your same situation differently. It may simply be the act of coping and healing if you've lost a loved one or ended a relationship.

Maybe it's a smaller thing, like fighting with a loved one or financial stress (not that those are small, just smaller than loss and grief). Whatever the case may be, you've changed and your body is like, "Okay, I've dealt with this. I'm good. I can keep going. I cried it out, and all my stuff is unclogged, so let's get back at it."

Breaking your physical and mental connection, as though emotions are just inconvenient nuances and tears and crying is just not important, will not allow you to physically have the outlet you need. Now, does this mean you have to cry at everything, every sappy song or movie or commercial, like some of us do, ahem, not naming names? No, everybody is going to be a bio-individual in how they experience, express, and feel their emotions. Some people may feel sadness and sleep or lay around and wallow, or feel really down and cry. Some will feel anger by getting flushed and shaky or not be able to speak or cry. Happiness may be felt by talking, laughing, and engaging with others, whereas some may just like the time to reflect and enjoy the calmness happiness offers.

We all have different ways of expressing our emotions, and

if we don't continually allow our emotions to be expressed, that physical energy is going to build up. They never get to express their creation. Anger's need for change isn't heard, so it can't promote the change it needs to promote. The energy from anger won't be redirected into a positive force of change, using your capacity to change with what's available to you right now and create a happier environment for yourself, which then creates more change and continues to allow you to heal mentally and physically. This helps you get to your weight goals with more energy to cook healthy meals and exercise more.

When you have residual stress from your work day, sitting in traffic, your relationships, or about money, you're never getting to those primary food areas that are causing that stress. Your emotions can't do their job either because they are constantly being re-engaged over the same thing and not being heard because we are trying to ignore them. "I just need to be happier and positive like all those motivational posters say." (I have a lot of those in my house. I like them, but I also know why they can be quite annoying at times.) That doesn't really come without doing the work of feeling your emotions and improving the primary food areas.

Feeling your emotions, going through a crying spell, talking through a conflict, or giving yourself an outlet to express anger doesn't necessarily mean yelling at someone or instantly telling someone you're angry at them. It's saying, "You know what, I feel angry right now and I have to go do something else and we can talk later." Take that anger, the energy for change, and change the situation. Walk away, go exercise, go drive in a non-road rage manner, but drive to reflect, put on music, watch a movie, take a nap, get grounded outdoors, spend time with a pet, talk to someone else. Do anything to change that moment. Then think about what your feelings are, what needs to be said. "Now, how do I respond to these feelings?"

When you cycle through that, you're giving yourself the opportunity to change, a way to feel that anger fully and recognize you can't just keep pushing off the anger and adopt a positive happy mindset of, "Oh, I'm suddenly happy all the time and everything is rosy perfect," when it's not. That's a form of denial and not productive. It is also another mentality for settling and not doing anything to change.

When you can feel your anger, do all those things I mentioned, or some, to try and let that anger out and know it needs to change. Something needs to change, and I have to look at how I can change. It's not about blaming and forcing others to change to make me feel better, it's about how can I change the situation. And with that, comes working in that positive mindset and then you get the happy positive mindset. It's the full benefit of working in the capacity of what you have, being the change you want to be, and engaging in happiness after you've felt conflict and reflected on those negative emotions.

It's really hard to say, "Well, I'm just not going to waste my time crying and I'm just going to keep going and be positive all of the time," and expect emotional growth and change to take place. Because emotional growth is not taking place, we're just setting things aside, not dealing with them, pushing them away, and choosing to ignore them by telling yourself you're a positive person. What we don't get to experience is the full emotional, mental, mind-body release of an emotion and then the renewed perspective of going, "Oh!! Sweet relief, I feel better now! I can keep going!" And sometimes, it's just a matter of endurance.

Like a marathon, in life, sometimes you've got to slow down, get a drink of water, and sometimes you have to do something. When you're in a hard, high stress time of your life—care taking, single parenting, financial struggles, or what have you—one bout of crying isn't going to suddenly remove all your struggles or stress, and likely, you'll cry again. But it's a coping mechanism and a way to get through it, and each time you are going to change, cleanse, and take all that gunk that's building up from all that stress and get it out. Crying is just responding, so you can keep going.

That positive mindset of living in today, enjoying people, and taking nothing for granted all comes by feeling your emotions. Being sad or angry by default doesn't mean you are taking things for granted. Hating your work or knowing your relationship isn't where you want it to be, or wishing for something different in your life doesn't mean you're taking what you do have for granted.

Taking for granted is not synonymous with feeling sad or angry about a given situation. I don't know how many times I've heard, spoken, or been told something along the lines of, "Well, you know it could be worse. Did you hear about [insert tragic story here]?" or, "Just when I think I have it bad, I heard this awful story of someone else's really hard times."

Yes, we should all be thankful for anything that we have that is going well or that could be worse. Absolutely. But don't use that to settle in to not excelling to the greatness that you can achieve for yourself. Don't use that as a means to stay put and not take risks or not want to change or hear the anger or sadness that is saying, "I need a change," because you can only experience what and where you are at right now.

You can have empathy and compassion and want to help other people who are suffering hardships and give to them. Don't use that as a means to stay put. And don't feel that wanting something more means you are unappreciative, taking things for granted, or are likely to have some terrible mishap soon to make you see just how good things were.

Also, this robs you of the true capacity to give to those other folks who are in need because you quickly become reabsorbed into being appreciate for what you have in fear of suffering loss, but it doesn't actually help the person who is suffering or make any changes for them. If you want to make sure you're being appreciative of something, be appreciative of what you have to give to help someone in times of hardship.

Continue to work on improving yourself and your life so you can feel happier and continue to use productive energy to give beyond yourself. Now, don't think for a second that being happy is easy. To be happy, you have to work hard because you are going to be changing and learning and growing, and you're going to have downfalls and times when you feel lost, defeated, or scared. Any underdog story will show you that.

I want to break down the core layers—you are at the center, your emotions are around you. Why is all of this important in a diet book? Because it's all about *you*. You are the center of your world, like the layers of the earth. In the very center core is you, your spirit, higher self, consciousness, or whatever you prefer, and this is surrounded by your emotions. Your emotions are what help you to interpret life, the day-to-day interactions with others, to help you decipher what's good, bad, safe, or scary. These emotional responses around your life events will help you to establish your belief system.

Your belief system has a pretty big job of keeping you on track within the areas of safety and "supposed to do's" while finding the good things over the bad. This often leads to the reduction of unpleasant feelings by any means necessary, so risks, rejection, or failure become things to prevent. This means you begin to believe your own internal messages and experiences as well as external messages.

Our belief system is pretty deep rooted in what we do, how we live, and who we surround ourselves with. Eventually, your beliefs align with what you believe you are capable of in life based on the emotional experiences you've had and the protection you form around scary or unwanted emotions, and your openness toward safe emotions.

Your comfort zone is formed which guides you to the safe options—the options away from anything that'll stir up any unwanted feelings or emotional response. What you are able to do is based on your beliefs, which is based on your emotional standing and experiences about life, yourself, and all of the things you've experienced thus far.

The emotional cycle is complicated to navigate and it can be hard to figure out what to do when having unwanted, highly emotional experiences. I don't like vague concepts. I like clear, concrete steps of action to give me something to do or use.

- Recognize
- Express
- Change

Recognize your emotional responses that require the energy to change and are usually also uncomfortable.

Express the emotion for yourself. Stop yourself in the situation and express it for yourself, which doesn't mean instantly yelling at someone when they make you mad. It means express the energy around the emotion. When you're angry, you have energy tied to that feeling. Your blood pressure may rise, your heart rate may increase, you may get hot and flushed, you may want to cry. You have to express that energy somehow to change the situation. So how can you change the situation?

By leaving. You tell the person you can't talk right now. If you're working with a difficult person and can't literally leave, ask for help from a colleague to step in. Do anything to change *yourself* in the situation. Also, remember to actually do this. Talking it to death isn't going to change the situation instead of getting up and changing the situation. I want to keep talking because I feel like that will help it, but most times, it doesn't. I need to say my piece and move on and then I need to take the energy from anger and let it change by expressing my emotions while working out, journaling, going for a drive, or any of the other activities I mentioned earlier.

Change. You're the action for change. Is this something that upsets me all the time? Well, then I need to do something. I need to be the change I want to see. I need to realize I am feeling these emotions and I am setting the pace at which these emotions are happening. I need to ask for help, get support, change jobs, end a relationship, go back to school, move to a new town. I need to learn how to treat myself better by eating better. I need to get more medical attention, or whatever the case may be, I need to take the steps to put change into place for myself, be it little or small. Take action toward the situation by fixing the primary food imbalance or deficiency that needs attention.

This is about you. This isn't about anybody else. It's not about their need to change so you can change, or that your employer does all these awful things so they need to fix it all. Yes, you can bring your needs to other people's attention and have an adult conversation, but if or when things aren't going to be remedied, then it's time to make another change. Keep in mind, even if you talk through your needs with someone else, they may or may not get met, but even if they do, it may not be enough if you still haven't made your own changes.

Boom. You're good. All of this process is what helps to create your positive mindset, the positive mindset of operating within what you have and do not have. You are going to explore all kinds of options and that also means recognizing if you have feelings of anger or sadness. This is the sparked energy for change and we need that to get to happiness. We need that to get to the end point.

Remember that when you start feeling like crying is pointless or if you're used to putting off crying, when you begin to engage and express your emotions, you may first start crying over a lot of little things and feel completely silly. Let it out. You likely have a lot of residual back up that needs to come out. Once you give yourself permission to let it be released, your body may be like, "Oh, yay! Let it out, let it out! Let's cry over every-thing!"

Then, after you level out a little more and let yourself cry when it comes up, it's no big deal. You're no longer wasting all this energy on *not* crying. This is something that has been conditioned into a lot of us from a young age because we are all raised to perceive the expression of our emotions, and we're all exposed to so many different messages at home, in school, through media, by our friends and so on and it's a lot of mixed signals. There's no one uniform way to handle, express, or talk (or not talk) about our emotions. Men and women are treated differently with what emotions are more acceptable for each gender to "have" or not.

So there's a lot of baggage there on how to express our emotions. I just look at it as plain and simple, we are humans, we are wired this way. Emotions are a part of life and our life experiences, they're part of our needs and survival. Let's deal with them in a productive manner and use them as tools instead of something to be ashamed of or to fight off and treat like they're wrong. As we continue to let these emotions cycle through us and come and go as they need to, we're going to become more even keeled. You'll improve these primary food areas and have even more energy freed up to focus on other important tasks that seem to be overlooked most of the time.

It won't be a big deal to get to the gym when you feel less stressed and exhausted by emotional damning. It's no longer such a huge task to cook a meal and let your kids help in the kitchen because you're not still fighting that anxious energy that has nowhere to go, so you feel less angry and can slow down and enjoy these tasks more often.

You will have more of a calm mindset to the do the things, big and little, that you need to do to take care of your mind, body, and spirit. The lack of release of a physical feeling around an emotion is going to build and it's going to create a physical expression of that emotion. When we're happy, we laugh, we cry, we jump or dance, or we just feel good. Or, maybe we get butterflies in our stomachs and shake with happy nervousness. When we're scared or angry and a situation is upsetting, we flee, fight, eat! Do something to make it stop!

We have physical responses to emotions which tells me if they don't get engaged and are shut down, they are going to stay somewhere with us. So we want to continually cycle through our emotions to avoid this from happening because the energy around these unexpressed emotions will create an internal parade of Gizmos and all his water induced cousins running amuck in your mind and body, looking for a way to escape, create, and do what emotions do, make change.

– five –

Call to Action

This next exercise will give you a visual, and help you find a new way of looking at these different primary food areas in your life to get a better feel for your satisfaction levels and how these are impacting one another. I have added some more in-depth questions for each one of these life categories to reflect on after it is completed.

If your image looks like a poorly made dream catcher, rest assure that's pretty normal. That's exactly how mine looked the first few times I did this. I encourage you to come back to this regularly and add in new dots as these areas continue to improve.

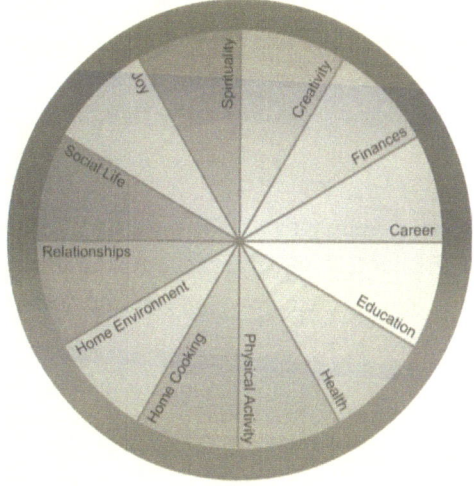

What does YOUR life look like?

1. Place a dot on the line in each category to indicate your level of satisfaction within each area. Place a dot at the center of the circle to indicate dissatisfaction, or on the periphery to indicate satisfaction. Most people fall somewhere in between (see example)

2. Connect the dots to see your Circle of Life.

3. Identify imbalances. Determine where to spend more time and energy to create balance.

© Institute for Integrative Nutrition | Used with permission

Remember, your life is a story or a movie, and even if it's only for your viewing, what do you want to fondly remember and what do you want to excitedly look forward to each day? Now, are you doing anything to make that happen, or are you overwhelmed in the everyday little things that bog you down?

Just as I encourage folks not to take on too much too fast with making healthy food choices and changes, I do not want you to take on too much too fast in changing your life. Nor do I want this to feel like some kind of exercise to see another way in which you are failing. Rather, this is laying the groundwork to know what exciting things you get to do for yourself.

Look at the area calling to you the most. It may be the easiest fix or the hardest, which is the most draining. If you feel completely lost, let's see how you can find some answers on your way.

Here are a set of questions to coincide with each area of the Circle of Life exercise:

(Spirituality, Creativity, Finances, Career, Education, Health, Physical Activity, Home Cooking, Home Environment, Relationships, Social Life, and Joy)

1. How do I feel about my... (creativity, finances, career, education, etc.)?

2. In what ways would I like to use or improve my...?

3. When I think of _____,
   I feel _____.

   Ex: When I think of creativity, I feel that doesn't describe me at all.

   Ex: When I think of finances, I feel tense and stressed because I'm so broke.

4. How would I like this area or primary food to change?

5. What am I able to do to ignite this change?

6. How are these different areas affecting my overall mental, physical, and emotional health?

7. How am I investing in my self-care and wellbeing?

This is not something you have to have all the answers for right away, but do take some time to jot down some notes or thoughts (in the book, on a paper or napkin, text yourself, however you like. Or talk out loud to yourself, just think and reflect on it in some manner.)

Understanding these realities of your life and being able to improve these areas to meet your needs is vital to making improvements in life *and* being able to break away from those unwanted behaviors, such as craving and turning to junk foods for entertainment or comfort.

Creativity. Often, this is only associated with artistic ability. I remember one time when I was a kid, my friend and I sat in art class, we were young, I don't know how old. She asked me who I thought had the best art projects and I told her she did. I don't recall if I actually thought it or if I was being nice. Eventually, she told me she thought my art projects were the worst in the class and I agreed with her, probably in instant defense to protect my feelings and also because they weren't very good. I was so not a fan of working with clay and drawing with markers on construction paper. To this day, still makes my skin crawl.

Nonetheless, something about that must have stuck with me somehow, not because she was a meanie or anything, we were kids, but the feelings I already had around my artwork not being good nor enjoying the types of art we were doing stuck with me as I never really engaged in those types of projects until I was in my twenties. I decided to try painting or creating some wall décor for my first apartment because I was tight on cash and if I was going to spend some money on wall art, it seemed more fun to make it than to buy it. In time, I developed quite a knack for painting abstract art and actually sold many of my canvases to friends or other folks who stumbled upon my work. Most importantly, though, I *enjoy* it, the actual act, the freedom of pushing paint around on a canvas and just watching the colors move into their own rhythm.

But there are *many* ways to engage in creativity.

Many people tell me they aren't creative at all because this is often associated with artists or crafty people, and if you don't or can't do these kinds of things then you aren't creative. I disagree. My husband, for instance, tells me he isn't creative, yet he can build computers and is a talented woodworker. He builds things and has a great talent for understanding how things work, and can repair things around the house, and has a talent for taking a complicated concept and explaining it in a way for others to understand. He is creating something–that's plenty creative to me.

Your creativity is specific to you. It may be in hobbies, in your work, in your lifestyle, your cooking, anywhere really.

What about your financial standing? This is a biggin'—wait, who am I kidding? These are ALL biggin's! Are you strapped for cash or doing well with money? Do you always fret and fear money will disappear as soon as it comes in? Do you disengage from it, let your spouse, parent, or partner handle the bills? Do you overspend? Or are you the opposite, always chasing the next raise, the higher income, and though you are good with money, there always seems to be the *next* goal as soon as you get the first?

Do you have healthy spending habits for yourself and your self-care—not overspending, or indulging in empty impulse buys, investing money in yourself with the quality ways in which you want to spend your time and on what you really want. Think about this carefully because we trade our *time* for money. If you are trading your *time* in an unfulfilling profession, your income may be spent in similarly unfulfilling ways. I've read many a stories of folks who make six figure incomes, still live beyond their means, and have all kinds of "stuff," but are stressed to the max, overworked, unhealthy, and still looking for more. Even with a high paycheck, you can still be broke, and even with a small paycheck, you can still be financially stable.

An interesting thing has happened for me over the years. I used to go shopping and yearn for all the things I couldn't buy, or I'd overspend to scratch some itch while working in my purposeless jobs. I now find myself in an entirely new place. I love my work, I don't dread Monday mornings, I know I'm doing something that not only makes a difference for others, but it makes a difference for me.

When I go to a store now, the "stuff" is cool, fun to look at, and sure, there are some things I want or will pick up that moment and purchase. But more often than not, I can calmly walk away, think about it, and not overspend. Despite the fact that I make more money, I don't find the need to just quickly spend it on this or that.

It's as though because I earn my money in a quality manner now, it should be spent the same way—on quality purchases and investments.

Education. Though it is often pursued for professional gain, this is super important for personal satisfaction. Sadly, many people go to school for something they aren't really interested in but feel is *responsible or safe*. First, education takes place all around us each day—sitting in traffic, working, engaging with others, you always have an opportunity to learn. Second, each one of these items ties into and shapes the next. Education can ignite personal growth, enhance your professional path, and increase financial circumstances, but also ties right back to creativity, may improve your personal level of joy and even your social life when meeting fellow students.

Do you see each item in this circle playing into the next? For instance, cooking may tie into your social life and your sense of creativity by hosting a dinner party and having friends each bring a dish while you cook one as well. Or you may find that your desire to play sports or attend a fitness class allows for healthy physical movement while also meeting new people or getting outdoors, allowing for a bigger spiritual connection while out in nature and getting a workout.

At the very essence of this circle is you. You and your inner wisdom—each time you try something new, find something you like, learn something different, you get a piece of yourself. Sure, it is easy to say, "Yes, this book/diet/class/church/friend is exactly what I've been looking for. This has done so much for me." But *you* have been looking for it, and your inner wisdom is what prompts you to engage in said "something" further because it may be just what is needed. Even when you make a mistake, your inner wisdom is trying to get through somehow, and learning to trust yourself will help you pick yourself up and move on to try again. Sometimes, to know which way you need to go, you need to go all the other ways just to be sure.

I like to think of it like trying on clothes—not always a fun experience but neither is returning your clothes back to the store, so we do it anyway. Often, when I put something on that is super cute on the hanger and super awkward on me, I hang it back and am ready to find the item that is great on the hanger and even better on me. And if I don't find anything, well, that's money that must be meant for something else.

Traveling a new direction in life is just like going to the dressing room to try something on. You may come out fabulous, ready to rock, or you may come out with feelings of defeat (and messed up hair). Either way, you don't want to be walking around naked or in outdated outfits your entire life, do you? Probably not because it's *uncomfortable*.

Walking around out of balance with yourself in these various areas of your own livelihood is like walking around out of style or naked–totally awkward or vulnerable feeling because if you aren't in touch with yourself and inner wisdom, who can you really count on?

I can remember, at a young age, being so excited to get asked out on a date. There was something so nice sounding about having a boyfriend. Oh, sure, I sound like many kids who want to have a boyfriend or girlfriend, I know. But that continued for me for years. It was one of my biggest primary food deficiencies. The next was an overall lack in self-esteem. For me, it was never a question of *if* I wanted to settle down, get married, and have a family. It was a matter of when it would happen and meeting the right person. Some primary foods will be so high on your radar that you may adopt a bit of tunnel vision in that you won't see or be concerned with others, and that's okay.

There is not one set process that'll work for everyone here. Each of you will your own path in improving your primary food areas. As I began to improve my relationships and my career, other changes in life became easier as well. For instance, making huge changes in my food choices was much easier when I had other positive areas of my life in place.

Just as your primary foods overlap and impact each other within you, the positive changes you can make with your primary foods will provide more momentum to continue making changes in other areas, and you never know when one change will bring about another.

I never thought that by learning more about healthy eating, and in turn, cooking would lead to potential income earning by holding private cooking sessions out of my home. And I did it with real approaches to cooking—smoke alarms go off, things are spilled, and sometimes I'm missing ingredients. Why? Because, likely, that's what will happen for my clients. We always have fun, so not only am I eating healthier meals, I'm cooking more at home, learning more skills, increasing my satisfaction, *and* getting the opportunity to earn money sharing these same skills and lessons learned.

Start with one area to begin making changes or improvements. Yes, this will take time, you will have to do some work and stretch your comfort zone, but it is doable. Even if you only have a few minutes each day to work on a goal of yours, each step you take will add up.

six

Road Blocks

Roadblocks are present for all of us, no matter what the task at hand may be—weight loss, saving money, meeting new people. Each of us have our own road blocks. Some are internal and some are external, but they are real for each one of us. Roadblocks are obstructions and will keep you moving forward. Roadblocks are what happens when all your worries, doubts, and fears are allowed to be in the driver's seat all of the time, and every potential mistake spells disaster or failure, which often seems to be one in the same.

Failures, mistakes, and unwanted outcomes happen no matter what, so what's the harm in going after your dreams? We all either do this to ourselves or have the certain someone who always has to warn you about all the risk, the hard work, or the potential heartache of failure involved in doing something outside your safe, cushy comfort zone. These external and internal influences become your roadblocks.

Are your roadblocks people you know or your own inner doomsday prepper? Are your roadblocks locked into your external areas of insecurity, say around financial security or social interaction with others? Or, are they your own internal feelings of self-worth?

For instance, I have roadblocks that are disguised as other people I know personally, and I also have a really overactive inner doomsday prepper! "What? You're doing what?? You may FAIL! You can't do that because it's not practical! What do you mean you're writing a book–what if NO ONE READS IT?" I imagine this voice being a lot like Jim Parson's character, O, from the Disney movie, *Home*.

Roadblocks lead to being talked out of (by yourself or others) doing something you may really want to do. I've learned from my own personal epiphanies that most of the time, when someone else is warning, explaining, or telling you something, they are seeing some element of their own actions in yours and are really speaking to themselves.

Now that you have your circle of life complete, we need to expand on this a little bit more. You're going to need three pieces of paper (or a large notebook-ha!) to complete these next exercises.

First page: Write down your top priority primary food items—you know, those big tickets in the areas from the Circle of Life exercise and the four areas of primary foods: career, relationships, physical activity, and spirituality. What are the ones that are the instant, "I want to improve these now," tunnel vision items?

It may be falling in love. It may be traveling, getting your Ph.D., having a family, or being on television. These are the really big life experiences that require the energetic determination (this to be discussed soon) to continue to pursue the experiences you'll be fondly remembering one day. How do these items tie in to the Circle of Life items you are finding deficiencies within? How can you improve your Circle of Life by chasing these big ticket items?

Get the second sheet of paper and fill it front and back, up and down with every single excuse, fear, doubt, and insecurity you have in your mind. Whatever makes you feel incapable of accomplishing these goals or improving these areas of your life.

Excuses left unattended or reasoned with for too long grow into roadblocks and then seem impossible to surmount. Excuses are really instant ways at processing *your* reality and making snap reactions to it. Excuses look at your past, your current situation, and potential "what if" unknown areas of life, and create all of the reasons why something is the way it is, or why something is not likely to happen or hard to do.

Congratulations. You have just outlined your first hurdles to your goals and identified your guidelines for moving forward.

We will start with the first order at hand that most of us share—our own inner voices and the voice of others. For self-preservation purposes, all of us are wired to stay safe, but what is safety when your personal safety is met and you're discussing the ideals of living up to your own true self?

Each person has personalized lenses in which life is experienced. It is extremely difficult to remove these lenses and all of the emotions tied with it because it is part of how you have experienced your world and life thus far.

It's really difficult when someone you care for is making life choices you see as unsafe, that'll draw unwanted social attention, potential financial strain, or other types of failures because you want to protect yourself and those you care about. Being on the receiving end of naysayers telling you what you should and shouldn't do, what's right or responsible, can be downright exhausting and limiting.

Don't give your own fears and insecurities, or others', any more power than what they deserve. See these feelings for true feelings, but also not always logical or the only considerations when looking at your life choices.

You can begin to recognize these are shared fears and you're seeing a glimpse of their own fears, doubts, and insecurities. Our fears can become so big and all-consuming that that it is even uncomfortable for anyone around to not follow the status quo.

It happens so naturally that we don't realize we do it, and it's often felt as though it is coming from a *good* place because others just want what is in our best interest and our best interest is to be safe. It's common practice for people to project their own fears, internal frustrations, and other feelings onto others. It's part of what we do and it happens often without us even knowing it. I've been the naysayer or the one to speak up in other's lives, and I've been on the receiving end of it, and, really, both sides are no fun, and both waste valuable energy being in opposition instead of in support of others and yourself.

Each individual has to overcome their own challenges and no one in your life, not the naysayers or anyone else, is bad or wrong for having these feelings, even when their worries come out in anger or judgment. After all, think of you how feel when you're hurt or worried about someone and feel as though there's not much you can do about it. We get angry from fear. Or maybe they are dealing with their own anger and jealousy at the thought of someone else going after big dreams in life when they are still playing small. Or the fear of going against what is socially expected of us and not being "normal."

Do you give your naysayer a voice? What if that someone, or many people in your life, haven't actually *said* anything to you that sounds like their true opinion, but you just *know* they are thinking it or don't agree with your choices. Don't give them a place to take hold and become a road block because even their opinion has no stopping power over you and what you choose to do. Most importantly, don't give your roadblocks an external face of someone else in which to get angry at or to feel stopped by or something to have to fix by gaining approval of external areas first before moving forward on your own path.

Begin to recognize this for what it is—just human nature all around many different faces of fear. Once you remove the conflict around these feelings, and remove the need to prove or yell or blame others for feeding your roadblocks, all that is left is a lot of energy to focus on change and the realization that you are empowered and able to either continue living in fear and play it safe, or step on out there and trust yourself to keep on trucking no matter what happens.

At the end of the day, you have to live your life, and you can thank these folks and your own doubts for their concerns and *use them* moving forward, but that means you make educated choices. It doesn't mean you have to, or should, sacrifice your personal goals or dreams in life.

I mentioned that fear is not the only factor to consider, and often times, it has a limited scope of vision but often gets put in the driver's seat because, surely, that's the *only* way to stay safe.

Yet, when you're scared, do you freeze up, get flustered, unsure of how to act or what to do? Do you want to hide or retreat, but ultimately get somewhere to *stay* safe? Right. That's the purpose of fear.

We have more tools and abilities to avoid unwanted outcomes, and we have the ability to surpass unwanted outcomes even when they do happen, so why does fear become the main driving force? This is something I am still working through in my own life each day.

Take the next blank piece of paper and write a thank you letter to your excuses and fears for being present to guide you away from unwanted results and wasted time, to remind you of what you already have and value and don't want to lose, and to shed light on those things you can stand to move away from. Write to all of the people in your mind who are secretly, or not secretly, betting against you and thank them for their concerns and their love for your wellbeing. You do not have to prove or get anyone's acceptance directly from them, contrary to movie and television show conflicts, which are solved quickly and in a few well written lines, you may spend a lot of valuable time and energy trying to convince someone of your own ability when you should just be doing things instead and letting actions speak for themselves.

What other excuses are there for you? For me, it was always time and money on the surface, but it was more about what I felt unable to accomplish, and I used time as a roadblock.

Even ten minutes of time can be contributed to one small step toward something that really matters to you.

Include in your letter that you will use the time you do have and you will find a way to be mindful of any financial investments you may need to make to pursue these parts of your life.

Once you write this, you can keep the thank you letter and that will serve as your safety net as it encompasses all the feelings around fears of yourself and others. It gives your fear a place to be and to be heard, but not to be the driving force in all of your decisions.

The list you have with all the excuses by themselves can be released. Recycle it, get markers and color a pretty picture over it, fold it into an origami craft, whatever you do, just know it's okay to not let these always be front and center. Your ability to recognize and avoid risk and danger will still be there if you allow someone else to take the driver's seat.

Now, take that first piece of paper with your big ticket items and all over this paper, front, back, and everywhere, write all of the emotions sparked when thinking of these things: joy, hope, happiness, pride, adventure, excitement, accomplishment, peace, education, growth. Put this somewhere visible, frame it like the first dollar earned, or carry it with you in your wallet. Or make it into a beautiful piece of artwork with colorful lettering, or again, an origami craft, or something that reminds you of what you are working for and why.

At the end of the day, those voices, outside influences, and your insecurities are yours. Your roadblocks will likely be similar in each area of your life—failure, making the wrong choice (whatever that means—we're just trying things on, remember?), no time or money, etc. If you are able to navigate or remove your roadblocks in any area of your life, you will be able to start removing these roadblocks in any other area of your life as well.

"But if I don't listen to fear and if I make the wrong move to try and accomplish something—what if I fail, or what if I make it worse?"

"Well, this is just my reality and there is nothing I can do about it."

"Other people just don't get it–bet she's had it really easy."

Roadblocks are stubborn. They aren't just going to disappear. They have needs and voices that should be expressed often, which can take up a lot of your energy because feeling this way begins to feel pretty close to having your own inadequacies or failures by all that you can't or are not doing.

So, one small step at a time. Say you want to exercise more but feel that it's kind of pointless to only do one workout at a time because it doesn't amount to anything. But it does. It's one small step toward creating a new habit in your life. It's one accomplishment for the week or the day or the month and it can't be taken away. If one missed workout is bad, well, then one completed has to be good.

And one missed workout is only *one time*. It's funny, isn't it? One workout to get started doesn't count because after doing it, you look the same even though your body aches in areas you didn't know you had, and your muscles are throbbing and you *feel* you should look buff, but you don't. So, surely, one time here or there doesn't do much. But when you miss a session, oh, world, lookout! It's the end of the freakin' world, and "I always do this, I start and then something comes up and I fall off the wagon again."

Stupid wagon. Forget about it! Your roadblocks and excuses and all the worries around this or that outcome—let it go. Just do your best for today and tomorrow is tomorrow. Every act of kindness and self-care and engaging in your best self is not wasted, doesn't matter how big or small a feat it is or how often it happens.

Roadblocks are yours—you own them. Heck, you've built them around what others have told you or what you have started telling yourself. They are yours to be torn down, remodeled; you can have detours to each of them. It just happens in life, some are more bogged down by them, and some are not.

Remember, in your thank you letter, the idea here is to thank these feelings or thoughts for what they are protecting you from or sharing with you, for being part of your life and knowing they'll always be there when needed. But now, it's time to look beyond all the same messages we get from them and see what else is there to learn from.

This is not about blame, nor am I saying it is your entire fault. This is about your own personal empowerment and the opportunities that lay right within you. No one knows your roadblocks as well as you, nor does anyone else hold more ability to affect your life more than you do, but you most certainly can have amazing love, help, and support along the way.

As you take one little step toward your goals, around your roadblocks, you're doing exactly what you need to be. Your goal is not just your end result but the experience of obtaining it. Just go for it and know each day that you are working to be one step closer to your dreams, and along the way, you will learn more about yourself, what you are capable of, and have a heck of a lot of fun.

One of my biggest primary food focuses was meeting a great partner to have a family with. As for romantic relationships, I was a habitual online dater. I actually met my husband online, and despite the many frustrations with online dating, heck, dating in general is exhausting, I continued to get at it and go again because I knew if I did nothing, I'd have nothing to show for it. I had multiple people tell me all kinds of things like, "You probably won't meet anyone that way. Why don't you get out more?" or, "I don't think there's anyone good you'll meet where you're at. You should probably move," or, "You're a little bit picky."

But I did what worked for me and I refused to settle because that's not fair to the other person nor to me, and eventually, I met my husband and started building the kind of relationship I had always wanted.

Sometimes the roadblocks are fed by empty indulgences, say for instance, overspending or seeking instant gratification instead of quality things that really matter, leaving you on an up and down, "I need something new," rollercoaster while also keeping you broke or strapped for time. Again, all of these areas continually shape and impact the next area in your life with you riding around at the center.

Being stopped by your roadblocks in life leaves out most of the excitement, opportunities, experience—all of that comes from getting out there and experiencing life for yourself in whatever ways you want.

If people were to give up on venturing down some path because of hard work, unexpected challenges, and all that comes in between, how boring would life be?! Likely, we'd have no Olympics, athletes, artists, or other forms of entertainment. We might not have transportation, computers, or any of the other modern day conveniences we enjoy. Heck, forget parenting! The truth is, when doing something new, your expectations will never be met. You have no way of gauging the outcome. Conversely, doing something you've done before, but with a new attitude, can have the same effect. It's kind of stating the obvious. Yet, we do it to ourselves and to others all the time.

Life is going to bring us challenges no matter if we are taking risks or not. Why not then pursue the things that'll bring us the most reward for the challenge? Most of the time, when taking on challenging tasks, venturing outside the familiar, taking on new opportunities, or just living life, we find that the hard work put out is well worth it, the learning and development that comes along the way is invaluable. Just because something is hard work and may be more than you expect, doesn't mean it isn't worth it. People work hard all the time at empty goals or for much less based simply on the social expectations of what *should* be done.

The question then becomes whether if what you are willing to work hard for is worth it or not to *you*. You can define your own success.

seven

Redefining Success

What does success look like to you? Is it measured by other people's responses to your accomplishments or just your own feelings? Is it measured by your needs or by the social image of success—money, beauty, happiness, everything those Jones' have? Or is it measured by what we have done or accomplished? Is it measured by the amount of pain and suffering and stressful times you've worked through? Is it measured by what you have earned versus what you were born with or into?

Can you be imperfect and make mistakes and still be successful? Can you be a successful artist even if you don't do it for a living? Are you able to be successful with healthy eating even if you aren't at your goal weight? Is it confirmed success when recognized by others, those closest to you, society, and your peers?

If you feel as though failing will let someone else down or that you will if you mess up at going after something you want will make you a failure in their eyes, keep in mind that you are much more than their perception of you and you know all of the details from the inside out. They only know it from the inside of their perception looking in.

Success is in the eye of the beholder. You can feel and be successful in your own way, and ideally, have people to celebrate with you not because all of your successes are the same, but because we should be celebrating ourselves and others a little bit more. Okay, a lot more, and tearing ourselves and each other down a lot less.

The pressure of dieting is often weighted by the level of success achieved with enough of the right kinds of effort. If you want success then you have to do *this* perfectly, and the better results you want, the harder you have to work. And you're only ever successful *if* you get the desired results that everyone expects to experience or that end up on magazine covers or gym ads.

Much like health, do we ever arrive at a place of success? I think we experience success, which is defined as a favorable result. I have experienced favorable results from changing the foods I eat on a day-to-day basis. I have experienced being able to easily maintain my weight without having to diet or count calories or really worry about what to eat. I have also experienced being addicted to sugar and processed foods and feeling lousy on a day-to-day basis because of it.

When it comes to dieting, success is often perceived as the final accomplishment that means you've arrived at the healthy destination of your goal weight. This means you are *only* successful if you reach your goals, and in order to reach your goals, you have to do it all. Right. Now. But if you begin to experience success, big or small, you can have a much more pleasant experience in making healthy changes.

The "suck-it-up-buttercup" mentality of suffer, do it all right now, and force it until it works because that's how we get results is a big cultural struggle many of us face. Redefining success will help you to be able to set clear boundaries for yourself and thus use your time more efficiently to take care of yourself and your priorities as well as those shared priorities for family, work, or any of the other hats you may wear. It also allows you the freedom to do things in your own way, which is super rewarding.

This pressure is why so many people get stuck in a cycle of self-defeat when we get off track by having one bad meal or a missed workout session. One may lead to two, and two may lead to three, and by three screw ups, well, heck with it all, if I'm going down, I'm doing it, man, and hitting the drive-thru on the way!

Redefine success as being each meal, each choice, right now, in the moment. You can be successful with each choice you make to love yourself. After all, if you eat a healthy meal for breakfast today and then have a not so healthy lunch, do you think your body rejects the nutrition from the food consumed at breakfast?

Body: Well, so much for that amazing breakfast, have to throw it overboard now because the cheeseburger is coming down instead. Maybe next time.

Guess what, you will get the value from healthy activities each single time you do something for your health, and each single time you do something, you increase the value it provides. Eventually, when you continually put healthy foods into your body, it becomes easier, and you'll find that the "bad" meals are less frequent than they may be now.

Being healthy isn't about arriving at one moment or place

of health. And this picture isn't the same for everyone. We have a form of tunnel vision in doing everything the same way, and if you can't do the right amount of exercise and the right kind of exercise and always eat the right way, well, then you won't ever get the results you want. This way of thinking, compartmentalizing each area of ourselves, health, and life is why so many people struggle—because what you need may be about something not even remotely tied to a nutrition lesson.

Each moment, each day, each interaction with yourself, others, and food can bring you healthy experiences and enhance your health. Each decision you make to nourish yourself means you are living a healthy lifestyle. Even a breakdown can lead to a breakthrough, so the "bad" days promote learning about doing better for yourself the next time around.

You don't have to be a super buff person who runs triathlons in the mountains while carrying twenty-five pounds of junk in a backpack, or eat nothing but tofu and greens to be healthy or living a healthy lifestyle. You *do* have to be making an effort to provide yourself with the nourishment you crave and deserve.

The Monday diet blues. Been there, done it many times, and hear it from others constantly. *Monday, I'm starting my diet, I'm going to the gym every day. No excuses, I just have to do it.*

This happens all the time and is said usually with feelings of anger or frustration. The best intentions are set, plans are made, internal mental exchanges happen, and game face is on.

Then, your co-worker pops her head in the office to see what your lunch plans are for the day.

Kelly: "You bring your lunch today?"

Me: "Yep. You?"

Kelly: "Yep," momentary silence while having the telepathic conversation that eventually reached our mouths.

Me: "I don't really want my lunch."

Kelly: "Me either. What do you want?" the glints of hope, of mischievous disobedience to the brown paper lunch gods, and the sweet satisfaction of rebelling against, well, I don't know what, but something.

Me: "Not sure, but I'm going on my diet Monday. After this weekend, no more. I'm going to bring my lunch and eat what I have, no matter what."

Kelly: "Oh, me too. So then, what do you want for lunch today?"

McDonalds was typically our go-to. One day, I remember sitting in the breakroom with our supersized meals, extra gobs of fries, and our fellow colleague walking in. Before he could utter a word of judgment about our fine binge fest, my friend says, "Don't say anything. I'm starting my diet on Monday," through a mouth full of Big Mac and fries.

He holds his hands up in the "don't shoot" manner.

"I mean, I have to have my Big Mac today because you know by the time Monday rolls around, McDonalds will go out of business, Budweiser will stop making beer, and I'll never get to have any of my favorite foods again!"

I nearly spit out my nuggets.

This cycle happened a lot for us, and eventually, we both started bringing and eating our lunches, mostly because we just got burnt out on all the other places. The all-or-nothing mindset is often said with a sigh of, "Well, I just have to do it. I don't have a choice." There's maybe anger and a few mentions of hope, or see what happens, or try harder, but there's not a whole lot of conviction or excitement expressed in this concern.

Focus more on the right now, each day. Don't carry the weight of the tasks you *should do*, but can't do it all right now—meaning, you can't complete five days of exercise now because you are only able to complete one day, so do that. This mindset is adopted and touted while not in the moment of temptation and other triggers for these behaviors, it's in the mindset of being angry at perceived failures, so of course, it's easy to feel strongly and focus on this sentiment. But without attention to the other surrounding causes, the cycle often repeats itself. This I know to be true from experience. But really, success can be experienced with each action you take toward your goals, be that with your weight and nutrition or in other primary food areas.

If you're thinking of exercising every day of the week and that's the only way to get results—I have to exercise every day of every week, at least so many times, in order to reach my goals, well, then suddenly, one exercise session becomes much more important when it is missed. "There I go again, failing at sticking with anything. What's the point? I'll never lose weight." But life happens, things come up, bad days happen.

Yes, if you want a certain looking physique, exercise can get you there, but it can come in all forms of physical activity, so why not incorporate more movement into your life for the sake of moving more? It can be something new each time or finding ways to be more active in your profession or on your personal time.

Success can be fun and it is not always about the results in the end. Think about the reality of doing something just to do it and learn. Success isn't about good or bad–though, in our culture that seems to be what it is all about. Good if someone else says so or if you're famous or earning money or lots of money for your work. Bad if you're the opposite of any of those things.

Success is about the act of setting your intentions around an action and then doing it.

That's it. That's what it is all about. The intention to do something–not to have the intangible goal of being at your goal weight, clothing size, or what have you. Rather, the intention to do the necessary action to create more income, or healthy eating habits, or better relationships, or more enjoyment at work, or love toward your own body as it is right now.

Your goals can be synonymous with action steps right now,

and success can be right here in this moment after each thing you do to live a healthy happy life. I am intending to take action and I'm intending this right now. I'm meal prepping today. Tomorrow's intentions are for tomorrow. And each act of intention contains an immediate start and finish and will contribute to changes I'll experience later down the line.

It's really hard to be motivated by long term results without any attention on the right now and the little successes you should be celebrating when you make progress each day.

Taking action to get healthy doesn't have to be dumping all the junk out of your fridge, loading up on fresh produce, and feeling as though you have to do *everything today*. I mean simply and intentionally take one step and accept one little step as being enough for where you are at right now. Accept these steps as success rather than, "I'll be successful when I reach my goal weight and then I'll be happy with myself."

There are people who find a certain way of eating or living and they seem to transform and become this new person after doing so. This is why it is so enticing to seek out the perfect diet plan. But I think there are many things taking place in this scenario—sometimes these folks find the diet plan they were already gravitating toward and this just put the pieces together.

Many folks turn this into a career and move on to write books, blogs, or recipes in the niche they find. Not only do they find a way of living suitable to their needs, but they find a new way to make an income doing something they feel passionate about and believe in. Also, for whatever the reasons, this is finally something they were able to do successfully–that, in and of itself, is a huge step forward in boosting confidence and self-worth, which will reduce stress levels and improve relationships in your life. All different forms of success, and all much more than just weight.

You can lose weight and still not be or feel happy. You can change your life, not your weight, live healthier, and feel happier. The confidence comes with the time and investment you put into yourself and your self-care. I think it is hard to treat yourself badly when you do things that make you happy.

Take the steps to get results to make you happy right now, which will bring happiness *and* desired results later too. You don't have to make yourself crazy trying to obtain a favorable result. In fact, what if you could also put forth a favorable effort to reach these desired results? Instead of forcing yourself to run on the treadmill, what if you found physical activity that actually appealed to you and worked with your schedule, skill level, and comfort level?

Redefining success for your present actions and future also means redefining success and failure of attempts in the past. You have to let yourself off the hook for any failures you may be carrying.

This notion that we all have one exact way to eat for good health can perpetuate the desperate need to fix and find something that'll work one magic solution. This is why weight loss failures are so much to carry on a personal level— because the ever eluding results are absolutely personal. I've heard stories full of anger and frustration surrounding the thoughts of, "I lost twenty-five pounds and gained it all back." I hear people refer to themselves as stupid, lazy, lacking will power, and many other colorful things. I also see that the weight gain always trumps the weight loss or any success they may have had.

You have to give yourself credit where credit is due. If you are carrying the self-loathing deluxe package of anger, frustration, guilt, and shame for having lost weight and then gained weight, please remember, you lost weight. You tried a plan, a routine, and a different way of eating, a product, or service. You lost the weight. Gaining weight after the loss is a separate occurrence. Unpleasant or angering as it may be, it does not mean you did not have the first success.

Use that as something to learn from and refer back to. And if you are reading this book, taking a class, or trying again, that my friend, is willpower and discipline. Just like the karate kid cleaning all those cars and painting the fence, though he didn't know it, he was learning something. Often enough, in order to trust our inner wisdom, we need to do things seemingly out of order, but it usually comes back to a good place of enlightenment.

My friend, you have many challenges you have to work through, many of which you may not have even recognized yet—unidentified, unique triggers to eating, out of balance primary foods, our coping habit of using food to medicate stress, sadness, happiness, and a variety of other emotions, and of course, easily available, cheap processed food which confuses our senses.

"I can't just let go of my mistakes. I have to be accountable to be successful and stay the course." Right. Accountability is supposed to help the cause, not perpetuate failure, but it is misused a lot and often confused with blame, shame, and other icky feelings.

You can be accountable *and* let yourself off the hook. These are two different concepts. In fact, beating yourself up for what you can't accomplish isn't holding yourself accountable either. Being accountable involves proactive measures, planning, intention, and action.

It also means realizing what outside factors influence part of your personal struggles. Each of us has our own set of struggles, and this is not about blame, this is about the ugly truth—we've all got baggage. This baggage definitely shapes the way we think, act, and perceive our life experiences.

It also impacts the food you eat, the way you live and spend your time, the people you spend time with, the relationships you have with others, and most importantly, with yourself. These hurdles are all part of you and impact your overall wellbeing. This isn't the point-the-finger-at-everyone-else-and-blame-them game, it's accepting the real world of processed, sugary food we live in. It's really hard to break away from this, especially when you feel everything is your fault.

Accountability isn't about punishment either. It isn't about comparing yourself to others or allowing others to pass judgment on you. There is an interesting relationship between our judgment of our own actions and the judgment we pass on others. I think we all are hard on others, whether we admit it to their face and actually say our true feelings or we think it, it is there to some degree. We judge others until we hear someone judge themselves.

As soon as someone reflects honestly about their feelings of anger or insecurity toward themselves, the other people around begin to pick up the pieces and help them work through it. Even if you'd been silently thinking the exact same thing before they opened up to you, suddenly, you feel bad for these slanted thoughts. The big difference being we don't often do the same for ourselves. We continually judge and shame ourselves without picking up the pieces and accepting the flaws, learning from them, and moving on.

In order to accomplish our goals, we often feel we have all these things "to do" and be first. You are enough right now. You are already where you need to be right now. I had someone say to me once, "Boy, I already have what I need right inside of me, don't I?" Wow. Powerful stuff.

You better believe it! You will go leaps and bounds in great directions when you finally listen to yourself, start living the life you want to live, and fulfill your needs. How much extra energy and time would it free up to just focus on taking one small step as you are right now toward your self-care. This includes loving yourself through mistakes, bad days, chocolate, and other hiccups. Not coming down on yourself for it or getting stuck in the blame-game self-loathing phase.

You are enough right now. Let go of the other stuff holding you down. Do this one step at a time. One day at a time.

eight

Energetic Determination

Before diving into the next segment of something that is super exciting to me, I must first explain how it came to be by addressing the bane of my existence—willpower. The social context of willpower is exhausting, and I don't know where the concept got so blown out of proportion, but I'll thank advertising for the weight loss industry because it suits all these companies really well to keep pushing their products and blaming failure on the users. Could you imagine if all computers, cell phones, or other techy devices blamed their consumers for not being smart enough to use the devices properly??

How can I work in the industry of health and wellness and cringe every time I hear the word willpower uttered? Isn't that the main concept of what I should be preaching? Nope. Willpower is an elusive mythical being like Big Foot or an uncreepy clown. It's treated almost like some superpower that not just *anyone* has enough of, but feels they should have enough of, and must carry the shame of not having enough.

You see, I often hear people mention willpower alongside being angry enough at themselves to finally make a change. The sentiment I hear in people's voices is full of frustration, guilt, or utter defeat. Most people say it with the sigh of hope, as though they are hoping to be graced with the presence of Ed McMahon or Hugh Jackman.

It's an overused term that is being dwindled down to a vague ideal only few possess and some learn to have. I can tell you that when it comes to making changes around my food choices, willpower wasn't the winning force for me. Primary food changes were taking place and my triggers to crave fast food were being dwindled and eliminated. Then, the simple act of learning about the clear connections I have with food and how I feel helped even more. In some respects, it really felt like the sweeter and "tasty" my life became, the more the empty calories foods began to taste awful.

Willpower did, however, happen to be the driving force behind me going to college and IIN, and driving myself to work each and every day despite hating every second of being there.

My husband and I sometimes have disagreements about willpower when it comes to diet and weight loss because he tells me he did have to use willpower. I am sure he did, and likely, it happened that way because his process for making changes to his food was different and his working life was in a better state than mine. That's interesting—the idea that we both use willpower, but in different areas of our lives. I had never really considered this before.

But what does that have to do with anything? It has everything to do with willpower and how we are using it in our daily lives to impact our health.

Have you ever thought of willpower as a muscle that is used on a regular basis every day? According to an article about willpower from the American Psychological Association, it very much is like a muscle that can be used and exhausted.

Todd Heatherton, Ph.D., of Dartmouth College, and researcher, Kathleen Vohs, demonstrated in their 2000 study, *Self-Regulatory Failure: A Resource-Depletion Approach,* how willpower is something that is used and depleted, so at some point in our day, we are not going to have enough willpower to cover all of our bases. In particular, one experiment was completed in which two test groups were asked to watch a sad movie. One group was allowed to freely respond emotionally and just watch the movie. The other group was asked to hold back on their emotional responses. After the movie, both groups were offered ice cream.

The group who had to stifle their emotions ate more ice cream than the other group.

Whoa! Game changer. Boom. The act of stifling our emotions and controlling our behavior requires willpower?! The subjects had to stifle their emotions for an extended period of time, so by the time the ice cream was offered, they had no more willpower left to turn down extra servings.

I wanted to jump for joy when I read this. Suddenly, I had a more profound understanding of this elusive, self-defeating broken record. This is why willpower always made me so sad—it was such a dream crusher to hear people with complete desperation centered around willpower to make changes in their lives.

Quoted from APA: We have many common names for willpower: determination, drive, resolve, self-discipline, self-control. But psychologists characterize willpower, or self-control, in more specific ways. According to most psychological scientists, willpower is a tool and this is how the tool works or should be utilized:

- The ability to delay gratification, resisting short-term temptations in order to meet long-term goals.
- The capacity to override an unwanted thought, feeling or impulse.
- The ability to employ a "cool" cognitive system of behavior rather than a "hot" emotional system.
- Conscious, effortful regulation of the self by the self.
- A limited resource capable of being depleted. (American Psychological Association. What You Need to Know about Willpower: *The Psychological Science of Self-Control*. APA, 2016. Web.)

Now, this makes sense to me. These steps are what you need to keep in mind when telling yourself to have more willpower, which are not just vague notions of being *good* enough or capable of withstanding temptation, rather it is an actual plan of action put forth to complete smaller tasks building to a bigger goal.

Another term I came across while reading up on willpower, courtesy of Merriam Webster's online dictionary, was *energetic determination*. I immediately loved this term because it feels so positive and full of possibility. What is it? Energy: capacity to do work. Determination: firm intention, resoluteness, stick-to-itiveness.

Break down these steps of energetic and determination as the capacity to do work with firm intention. This means what you are doing right now, regardless of results or outcome, regardless of shifting gears.

Now, if you think of the first step in will power as I've listed above, the ability to delay short term gratification by use of your capacity to do work with firm intention, how do you feel? Is that more clear than just saying, "I need to have more will power next time." Sigh. Groan, feeling defeated.

This to me offers clear steps, if you are doing work, you are doing something. That may be keeping busy when having a sugar craving by doing something else sweet in life. It may be reinforcing your intentions by writing your wants and goals down.

Use energetic determination to keep your momentum going, and apply that to the steps above to give you actual concrete methods or tangible ideas of what you can do to engage willpower as a muscle.

So no more forcing this vague notion of willpower? Can I get a woot-woot?! (Totally acceptable to fist pump with your wooting. No one is watching, go for it! And if you're out and they are watching, do it anyway and tell them about my book–ha!)

Energetic determination has conviction and motion, and it makes me envision someone actively seeking results or answers. Any creator, inventor, or person who has successfully reached a goal after many failed attempts didn't just force it, they had the capacity to do work with firm intentions. This energetic determination is what drives the star character in a movie to give it another go, whatever it may be. The music starts, the inspirational scenes begin to play out, and remember, "No one puts Baby in a corner."

Energetic determination is a commitment, not a whirlwind fling for this one. This is marriage, not a one-night stand. This is thick and thin, good and bad, ups and downs, make mistakes and then fix it. BFFs or bromances. Oh yes, this makes me feel good again.

It means we are in this together, for the good, the bad, and the in-between. It allows room for errors, imperfections, and falling of the proverbial wagon and saying, "Good riddance, who needs to ride a wagon anyway?" This is the same fervor I see in my toddler when trying new things—he just keeps trying something until it works. The thought of each failed attempt doesn't even seem to be present in his continual efforts other than to modify past attempts to be able to accomplish what he wants. Eyes on the prize the entire time.

From now on, when you think of willpower, you need to think of the above listed steps, the actions taken to use willpower as a muscle. Where are you already using your willpower and what ways can you reduce the willpower being exhausted in your day-to-day routine so you have more of it left over to pass up the drive-thru or make it to the gym or dance class.

This all ties into the other areas we've looked at. If you have imbalances or deficiencies in your primary foods, that is where your willpower is being drained, so now you have even more reason to get that straightened out. Over time, food will not be such a big deal, it'll just be food and you know what, more than likely, it'll always be there for you. (Especially the cheap processed foods!) Basically, what feelings food used to provide emotionally in quick short bursts, your new life experiences will give you the full spectrum of the actual emotions you are seeking. You won't want to binge on

Oreo truffle balls during your work day (not one of my finer moments.). Notice the want in there, that is key.

Energetic determination, just with health or success, doesn't require anything other than your own desire to try and keep moving, even if you aren't entirely happy or living your positive affirmations to the fullest. Over my many hours of reading, oh, so many self-help books, many seemed to have the same sentiment or prerequisite of being happy with yourself or in general.

Now, I was happy in that I didn't treat other people like crap, I was friendly, and all that. I didn't take things for granted, well, okay, I did, but tried really hard not to do so. But I wasn't happy in the same capacity these books were describing, and I always felt as though before I could even begin to fix the problem I was reading about, I had to first fix myself, change my attitude to something I just wasn't. It was always discouraging to me.

I read a book by Barbara Sher called *I Could Do Anything If I Only Knew What It Was*, and it was a game changer because she dives into this exact sentiment I was feeling. She gave me permission to be exactly where I was at emotionally, and to just do the work anyway. I cannot tell you how empowering this was because I had one less thing to beat myself up over—not being happy with the lack of direction in my life. That meant I could focus on the problem at hand, and for me, at that time, it was figuring out what the heck to do with myself professionally because I was exhausted from working too many jobs I didn't like.

I am going to tell you the same thing. Wherever you are at

emotionally, you do not need to change it to get work done. You just have to get work done and take one little step at a time. Energetic determination is about the momentum of continual movement from point A to point B, and your train is ready to leave the station any time you are.

nine

Back to Basics

Labels. We like to label Every. Thing. People. Food. Conditions or personality traits and types. It gets downright exhausting keeping up with each latest category and knowing which one you fall into. (Seriously, I have no idea if I'm a Gen Y or X, or XY).

We label things and labels have associations tied to them. I remember when a friend mentioned a local restaurant being a "hipster place" because they have gluten-free and vegan options. I was so excited to be in the hipster category for being gluten-free instead of the "you're a pain in the butt" club. Ha!

Seriously though, think about all the different labels around food—organic, non-GMO, kosher, vegan. Then there's the classics low-fat, low-sodium, sugar-free. And that's just a lot of the marketing descriptions used to market foods or food products to the masses. That's not even getting into all the various dietary theories catching attention. Generally speaking, in today's marketing mayhem around nutrition, we like to classify each food as either good or bad.

Nutrition is a very interesting area of science because many of the different dietary theories contradict one another, and somehow, most of them seem to work and have studies to back it up. From a professional perspective, I've seen this grow into intense disagreements about what is "right" or "wrong," and from personal experience, I've been just as confused, heck, sometimes I still am!

We want one answer. Surely there is one way we should all be eating and then we can stop waiting for the latest article or information on the most recently discovered super foods or diet. This is where the problem comes in. We are expecting there to be just one. (There can be only one! Nerd alert.)

What occurs time and time again is that one answer that worked for your best friend, co-worker, the actress on the magazine cover doesn't work for you. You try your best. Give it all you got, and it doesn't work for you, so what then? What does that mean?

Funny thing about food—for a long time, after eating, I'd get all phlegmy and constantly feel the need to clear my throat or cough or something. I felt like a really gross old man trying to spit up a hairball. Through some random chain of events, I think because I told a GI specialist I had difficulty swallowing, he wanted to do a scope down my throat to take a look-see. I thought, yes! Finally, you'll find this everlasting gobstopper like ball of mucus and can pull it out of there.

Wrong. They saw nothing that would indicate there was something going on in my throat. I was told on a follow-up phone call that maybe I had a case of globus pharynges, also known as globus sensation, globus, or somewhat outdatedly, globus hystericus, commonly referred to as having a "lump in one's throat." This is the persistent sensation of having phlegm, a pill, or some other sort of obstruction in the throat when there is none.

"So, basically, you're telling me it is all in my head then?" was my reply, and he confirmed. Somewhat insulted, somewhat on the verge of, "Well, I guess I can stop worrying about it then," I didn't try to figure out what this was anymore. But I always knew it was the most, uh, active, after eating and usually after eating junk foods. I thought perhaps my guilt was taking on the form of mucus.

I promise there is a point to this story, but now let me explain to you a bit of my professional background. My training was based on accepting all of these different theories as not to prove or disprove or promote one over the other, rather to get us to thinking, to challenge us. It was about the acceptance of many different ways people can get healthy and that as a professional in the industry, to remember to work with the individual first and foremost, and the tools to help your client come next.

We were challenged to hear contradicting dietary theories presented from the leading experts in the fields as well as sharing with one another, from student-to-student, what we personally experienced while trying different plans or theories to improve our own health and wellness.

This is not a natural or easy concept to implement into one's life or professional practice because we are often looking for the solid one answer to fit everyone's needs. As a student, it was even more frustrating to feel like, "Yes, victory is mine! This Ayurvedic-macrobiotic-vegan-paleo-raw way of eating is IT!" And then it doesn't work for my clients, or the next lecture given *also* makes a lot of sense and *also* feels like it could be IT.

When it comes to nutrition, there are some clear steps that are pretty basic and unify a common ground of the multitude of dietary theories on the market today. The rest, well, it's getting really complicated and heavy, but so are our lifestyles when it comes to our exposure to food, processed foods, high amounts of stress, continual cost of living increases, sleep deprivation, nutritional deficiencies, too much multi-tasking, and exposure to more and more screen time, pollution, and the list goes on.

The theory of bio-individuality encompasses all of these realities. It's means that one person's food is another person's poison. I didn't really buy into it right off the cuff. I mean, poison is a little much, right? Of course. But as I continued on my own personal path, making dietary changes, the more I realized this is very much a truth.

You know that phlegm issue I had and the supposed case of "it's all in your head?" Well, I don't have troubles with that anymore unless I eat certain foods. As I learned more about what foods were making me feel bad and what foods were working for me, many issues I had continued to clear up. Reducing my dairy, soy, and fast food intake pretty much eliminated the need to down a box of Mucinex after my meals.

You are likely aware of people with different types of food allergies to nuts, eggs, or shellfish, and these can be very dangerous, very fast. But what about when the exposure has an unwanted impact on our health but isn't quite as severe as those other allergies? What happens then?

Poison is a substance with an inherent property that tends to destroy life or impair health.

It's impossible to look at nutrition as all of these foods are good for everyone because we are all different. So what will make one person's health flourish may make another's dwindle.

If we were not in a time and place where food is mass produced and able to be shipped around the world, if we were all still eating local foods within a short proximity to where we live, what would that look like? Now-a-days, buying local is a bonus and often hard to come by. Heck, I don't even know what's indigenous to Missouri these days!

There are entire cultures of people who do not consume dairy products, yet dairy, by some, is touted to be a nutritional staple. People indigenous to cold climate areas consume high amounts of animal fats yet do not suffer with high levels of heart disease. Areas located by large bodies of water are going to live off of fish and plants from the water, whereas more landlocked regions will have other forms of livestock and plants to survive off of.

Now, though, with food being shipped all over the globe, and much of it being man-made in factories, some of which ship in specialty ingredients that are far from being indigenous to the final grocery store destination, it's no wonder people are getting super confused on what to eat and trying to find a simple answer of good vs. bad.

Healing with food is about learning how to nourish your mind and body by eating foods that will give you the vitality each day to live the life you want to live and learning what works for *you*. This is what the beauty of bio-individuality allows for–the individual and the ability to use and explore many different options of eating and healing with food.

Your body is an amazing tool and resource, and healing your body begins by working with it instead of against it. When you eat too much, you feel icky and bloated. You unbutton your pants and likely guilt yourself for having been "bad" yet again. When you eat foods that do not fuel your body, you'll feel exhausted. When you drink too much alcohol, you feel it, right? In all of these situations, you trust what your body is telling you and recognize it as a message to not do this again, and if you do, wait for a while, like for the next holiday season.

Because weight is one of the most common motivators for most of us to improve our food choices, it's often the only way in which progress is measured. There are so many more ways you can tap into the results of healthy food choices and its affects—your mood, complexion, digestion, anxiety, energy levels, sleeping habits, attention span, muscle aches and pains, or a variety of other little or big ailments.

You can learn to connect the dots of what is right for you by paying attention to the physical queues you are being given. I want you to remember this moving forward because it is key to being able to call your own shots.

I started out by reading ingredient labels and that was it. I gravitated toward food products that had ingredients I clearly understood or knew I would have in my own home. I didn't pay much attention to calories, fat, or other parts of the nutrition table.

I have battled neck aches and headaches for many years,

I've felt tired much of my life, and just didn't feel excited by much, just sluggish and heavy. After working with my chiropractor and applied kinesiologist for a few months, complaining about much of the same problems, he suggested trying something just to see what happens, and asked if I'd be willing to go gluten-free for a few days.

By the time I started working with him, I'd tried the prescriptions, physical therapy, other chiropractors and regular adjustments, changing my pillows, my posture, doing exercises, having lighter purses, wearing the right shoes. Nothing seemed to work. So, really, trying one more approach, that for all things considered, was really no big deal to do, was fine by me.

He suggested this based on the testing he had done from his techniques in applied kinesiology. While I know some may be skeptical of this or other alternative approaches, I'm a try-it-out-and-see kinda person. If it works for me, I'm going to stick with it. That's all I know. This is not my professional area of expertise, and this is my personal approach. Besides, by this point, I'd tried everything else. What did I have to lose?

After completing some tests, he had a few dietary change suggestions to make which were to eliminate wheat, dairy, and highly sugary items. I said, "Sure, and what is gluten and what can't I eat?" I did this with every intention of it being a temporary experiment...four and a half years later, and I haven't gone back to it.

After the first few days, I noticed something that was hard to describe. I felt light. That's the only way I can describe it. I felt as though I wasn't so heavy and sluggish anymore, having always been a small person, it was odd to always feel bogged down with weight, and this was a big difference. I also noticed in time, my lower belly became much more flat overall. I've always had the bloated lower belly, which I thought was a place where I carried weight funny.

From then on, I noticed relief with headaches, I felt more energetic, and didn't get as groggy or lethargic, unless of course, I was stuck at work staring at a computer screen, full of boredom. Then I could fall asleep with one blink.

This was a game-changer for me. So much of what I'd been experiencing for most of my life was improving, and it was the first step for me to really become in touch with the impacts food had on my body.

I didn't plan to test the waters again, but one day at work, I was stuck at a working lunch and pizza was provided. I figured it probably wouldn't be *that* big of a deal, and I couldn't get time to get out of the office for food.

Not only did the pizza taste like cardboard with a hint of white flour, within a couple hours after eating it, my head was spinning and aching. I felt like a narcoleptic, stricken with vertigo. It was awful! All of the little things I'd regularly felt over the years came back with a vengeance. It felt like the worst hangover I've ever encountered.

This was an epic turning point for me because prior to this experience, I did not have luck in kicking the fast food cravings. This was the first time I was able to rely on my body and began connecting the dots between food and how it impacted me. Because I now had a clear cause-and-effect from eating crappy food to feeling crappy, I just didn't want the food anymore.

This works *for me*. If I have even a homemade piece of bread made with minimally processed ingredients, I still get a dizzying headache, not to mention, it doesn't taste nearly as good as it once did. It's not a fad, it's not Celiac (at least I don't think I qualify in that category), it's just something I know to be true for me. Foods made with gluten don't sit well with me, and that's that. If it changes again one day, great, but for now, I'm good.

Does that mean I'm going to tell everyone I work with and who reads this book that they need to go gluten and 98% dairy-free just like I have? No. You've got your own healing process to go through, and treating everyone with the same specific approach doesn't interest me because you may be able to eat wheat or dairy without the same issues I have. (Sticking my tongue out at you now.) Nor is it what I was trained to do. I'm trained to look at you, the bio-individual.

As I continued implementing changes, I could easily identify different foods that would trigger headaches or other unwanted reactions and made modifications to my diet. If you had to classify my eating habits today, I'd fit closest to the Paleo Diet, which I completely stumbled into after making a series of changes. It was all because of going gluten-free and needing a new option for a wedding cake. I was at the local farmer's market and saw one lone tent selling gluten-free goodies. When I saw chocolate chip muffins, I was all for it.

Having ordered my wedding cake prior to going gluten-free, and then realizing I wanted to stick with it, I needed something else for me and my husband to enjoy, and turned out, they were able to come to my rescue. I learned they were paleo bakers, so when I wanted to bake, I knew that was an option for me for recipes. In time, and during my training at the Institute for Integrative Nutrition, I learned more about dietary theory and realized I liked and already ate most of the foods on the diet, so I began to use it as a resource for more recipes and meal options.

With each healing step I took for myself, I got better results, was able manage my weight, and discovered and cleared up more and more issues like a Candida overgrowth. Don't get me wrong, it was not always easy, and there were times I got to be like a dog with a bone and stayed really strict on dietary changes. That's easy to do, but in time, I recognized I was denying attention to primary food issues by focusing on improving my secondary foods—like I said, they are all connected.

Modern nutrition and the food industry is a mess. Seeing all the different kinds of diets, foods, and food products along with gimmicky diets or products is a lot to take in. Plus, you have finger pointing from different professional groups who all want to know the best way to get you healthy or thin, and belittle or point fingers at those who don't. There's a lot of "who is right" vs. "who is wrong" out there, and it is a lot of noise detracting from helping those find solutions.

Sometimes, truly healthful plans may often be overlooked or categorized in the same gimmicky category when that is far from the truth. One of the biggest hurdles is that we are, for the first time, experiencing all the fallout from decades of processed food consumption with the older generations who were introduced to it down to today's youth, many of whom, are overweight, battling diabetes as children, and will be climbing an uphill battle most of their lives just to get to what should be our natural starting point of optimal weight and health.

Food is our life source, and if to be used as our medicine, we must do so the way we use modern medicine—we need to look at the individual first.

Medicine is used for symptoms, but there's always attention paid to the individual—any other medical conditions, allergies, age, pregnant or not, etc.

So, then it would be clear to understand that if I have a certain set of health issues and another woman has a different set of health issues, the diets we should follow may differ from one another, right? Right. A young boy is not going to eat the same way as a pregnant woman or an elderly adult. Likely, you are going to crave different foods as well.

Bio-individual characteristics consist of age, gender, race, social class, blood type, medical conditions, and genetic history to name a few. Personal traits are inclusive of baggage. I'm not kidding. Seriously, we all have baggage, some good and some bad. Our baggage holds the life experiences and perceptions we have built, and this definitely affects our food choices, success with weight loss, and the process in which change can take place. It affects stress, how we process experience, and how we release our emotions. Everything.

This theory provides insight in the nutrition world as to why there are no hard and fast rules suitable for everyone, and why scientific studies are produced to back up multiple theories. But we are all still left wondering, "What the heck do I do?"

As a bio-individual, you will be able to learn the different types of foods that will make you feel your best. The best first step is to get more nutritionally dense foods in your body, which will be your plant foods. Add healthier foods to your diet each day, in any way you need to do it.

Then the next piece is to use your cravings to work for you instead of against you. First and foremost, when you have a craving for sweet or fatty foods, your body is likely looking for energy and your psyche is looking for the dopamine pleasure response from these foods to satisfy any stressors going on.

Did you know that you can get your body to send you cravings for healthy foods too? Yep. Your body is actually seeking energy and nutrition, but your mind and today's processed foods culture can make it easy for these messages to be drowned out or misunderstood as something different, especially if you've had many years of eating only processed foods.

So why not make it your nature to crave certain foods that work for you instead of against you. It is simpler than you think. You just need to give it time and stop worrying about perfection. You know, I'm a healthy eater and I can't tell you the last time I had a salad, which is the go-to healthy meal most people mention when dieting or being good. But I do have a lot of vegetables throughout my day. Simple example:

Breakfast: Bacon and eggs with onions and zucchini or radishes. I sauté veggies in a pan in oil or butter, scramble the eggs in a separate pan, and done.

Lunch: Open face sandwich with a little mayo, mashed avocado, mixed greens, and a pile of fermented sauerkraut on top. Check out the brand, Bubbies, for great fermented foods. These are loaded with healthy probiotics for our gut.

Dinner: Beef, fish, turkey, or chicken along with roasted veggies which may be cauliflower, broccoli, Brussel sprouts, asparagus, or a combination. If I'm really on my game, my burger will be wrapped in lettuce leaves and topped with more greens, but this doesn't always happen. Oh, and I'll add oven fries occasionally as well.

Butter. Salt. Pepper. Basic flavors. These are all okay to use when cooking. Get the fancy salt, pink or purple or red or whatever all the fun colors are. We do need salt, just not the refined stuff in the .99 cent shaker from the store that has nothing of any nutritional value left in it.

Yes, you can eat red sauce or dressing or BBQ sauce. Don't use a gallon of it, and as I mentioned before, it's about what you are ADDING to your daily food choices. Get in more veggies, even if that means they are skewered, painted with BBQ sauce, and thrown on the grill. Okay, fair enough. Done. Eat your veggies.

The veggies still provide nutrition if you eat them with junk food. It's about the amount of vegetables you are taking in. If your only intake is shredded iceberg lettuce at the sub shop, well, you likely don't need me to tell you that's not cuttin' it.

But if you eat a huge bowl of salad, since that's the go-to meal, and you use dressing on it, great. Eat your veggies. You will still get the nutrition even if your dressing is no good. Eventually, you will develop a taste for these foods with less and less fluff. I can speak from experience.

ten

Whole Foods, Zombie Foods

I remember the days when I would finish a meal and unbutton my pants to allow for the food baby belly to roam free. I'd feel just icky, and kind of like grease was coming out of my pores. Usually the guilt of overeating unhealthy food at the latest birthday dinner out or what have you would set in within minutes of the last French fry being consumed. I'd tell myself, "Never again. Monday, starting Monday," or, "Tomorrow, no more junk food." Of course, that only lasted for a short while.

While the food you eat won't actually make you a zombie in the dark comedy paranormal fantasy pop culture kind of way, you may have another experience while consuming nutritionally empty food products. They leave you feeling the effects of brain fog, lack of energy and mental focus. You're left yawning frequently, slumped over in your chair, staring at your computer or television or steering wheel, and replying to others with glossy eyes and a, "Huh? What are you talking about?" yawn, "Where's my coffee/soda/sugar?" At least that was me not too long ago.

Most of us have felt the effects of food hangovers from zombie foods. As I mentioned to you before, and I meant it, I'm not the type to dictate to my clients what they should or shouldn't eat. My husband (poor schmuck), yes, I tell him what to eat, even if he doesn't listen, I still mention it.

Because, well, I love that guy and he is helping me raise a family of little people, so I have some personal investment in his wellbeing.

With my clients, I simply want to provide education and resources for them to consider. At the end of the day, it is ultimately up to you to determine what you want to eat or not eat. Why? Because you need to be your own guide and you don't *need* me to tell you what to do. You'll be able to figure it out using your inner wisdom and by relying on?? You got it, your bod. Furthermore, as with anything in life, you have to want these changes and knowledge for yourself to see any improvement.

In today's world of modern nutrition, we are inundated with a crap-ton (that's a technical term) of information on ingredients, super foods, and everything in between. People don't know if sweet potatoes are carbs to be avoided or a nourishing food. It seems many folks feel they need to have a degree in nutrition just to know how to eat healthy. It doesn't have to be so complicated, but unfortunately, it is.

While I do think, in some manner of speaking, the intentions behind processing food may have been good, the unfortunate results decades later are that it has gotten way out of hand. We have become accustomed to eating food products for the basis of our daily meals with whole food items as a side here and there. Zombie foods are nutritionally empty and make you feel, well, like a zombie, or dazed and confused, or any variety of areas in between. Perhaps you have severe sugar swings which result in drastic mood swings, making you happy one minute and raging hungry the next, kind of like a zombie.

Are processed foods always bad? No. That is why becoming educated is so important. There are many packaged or processed foods that are okay to eat because they have minimal ingredients which are all recognizable and edible items. There are some food products that are healthy, but knowing which ones and how to make that determination will help you immensely.

Let us first look at the difference. Whole foods will vary based on who you ask because we all have a different idea of how much processing or refinement is okay. Typically, whole foods are defined as *food with little or no refining or processing and containing no artificial additives or preservatives; natural or organic.*

I consider fruits, veggies, seeds, nuts, legumes, beans, poultry, foul, fish, and red meat to be whole foods. These are easily identified because they are a complete food item that can be eaten alone and provide you with nutrition and satisfy hunger.

You can learn a lot about nutrition with a couple of simple steps.

1. Eat food that is an entire ingredient.

2. If it is a food product, read the ingredient label.

   a. Are you okay with the ingredients? Or do they make you think, "Hmm, I'm eating a science experiment. Maybe I shouldn't eat that."

3. Try different types of foods while reducing others and let the results speak for themselves in terms of energy levels, complexion, sleep, mood, hunger levels.

The simplest question to ask is, "Where is this food sourced?" Where did it come from? Was it grown, and if so, with what? How long did it have to travel before it hit your plate? If it is in a package or can, how was it made and what is preserving it? For any animal product, where did the animal come from? How was it raised? How was it killed? Regretfully, most farm animals are not treated in a humane way for the duration of their lives or during their slaughter. Shopping local, cutting down on portions, and knowing where your food comes from is very important in creating a healthy, balanced diet for yourself. This is a long process, so give yourself time to make one small change at a time. I'm still doing this myself.

Whole foods are food. It is what we once grew, gathered, and hunted. Our bodies recognize these items, even when our mind and emotional self doesn't, as a source of nutrition, energy, and nourishment. Our bodies use, break down, and digest these foods while absorbing the nutrients, vitamins, and minerals provided.

Back in the day, preserving food used to consist of adding sugar, fat, or salt to a food item to make it last longer. Now, preservatives are made of chemicals and we no longer simply have preserved foods, we have processed foods, or zombie foods, leaving us all malnourished, tired, and foggy. These may be found in vending machines, grocery stores, or any store for that matter, the drive-thru, etc.

Not sure if you have a zombie food or whole food? Here are some typical traits of a zombie food item:

- Long shelf life
- Does not mold or decompose (I still have a fast food

cheeseburger in a plastic bag that is over two years old now.)

- Lengthy list of ingredients
- Most ingredients are not easily identifiable
- Added sugars, salts, and/or fats

Most of my life, I fought feelings of sluggishness, anxiety, mood swings, UTI-like symptoms, headaches and neck aches, acne, fluctuating weight, a bloated lower belly, and trouble focusing or staying clear. I grew up eating many, many zombie foods.

Two things happen when you have a diet comprised of zombie foods. One, you load your system with unfamiliar gunk and you miss out on the micro and macro nutrients you need. (Fancy nutrition verbiage alert—all micro and macro nutrients mean are the big and little nutritional components of food. Micro would be the small items like vitamins and minerals, while macros are the big items like fat, protein, or fiber. Not necessary to understand the difference to eat healthy.)

I like to think of sorting through items given to you by friends or family for some reason or another that begin to accumulate over time. We keep them, thinking, "Surely, one day, I'll be able to use this." Then, of course, we have to find somewhere to store these items. And when all of these extras begin to take up too much space, we get the urge to clean and get rid of them all. Most times, I find myself thinking, "What in the world did I keep this for?"

By this point in time, there is so much stuff accumulated though, it takes a lot of time and effort to clean through it. It also can become a stress for some people, cluttering up their space or domain, which should be inviting and comforting.

Think of your body like your house, after all, you do live there, but you continually have all this stuff piling up that your body is trying to find a use for, but there's nowhere to store it. You will physically feel the stress of carrying these lingering ingredients and lack of nutrition in your body, resulting in lack of energy, mood swings, weight gain, or other physical reactions. By missing out on nutrition, you're missing the tools you need to function at your fullest potential every day.

For decades, calories-in and calories-out was the way to go. Today, it is much more complicated than that because it's no longer just about weight loss. Weight loss is the most sought after goal, but it is only one of many side effects from a lifestyle loaded with processed zombie foods. How exactly do our systems break down and process ingredients such as:

- Artificial sweeteners
- Artificial colors
- Enriched flours
- Other chemical cocktails

Studies are out. Studies are inconclusive or only completed on certain groups. Everyone has something different to say about what is good or bad. The driving force in purchasing different foods or food products is weight loss, and marketing has exploited this desire because it is not regulated by anyone, creating a product and packaging it in a manner with implications of weight loss is good enough. It is implied that the low-fat will result in weight loss or that low-sodium is healthier than regular because sodium is bad, right? So, with all of this marketing information that is dancing on the lines of being health advice, people who are just trying to eat some healthy foods and lose weight are totally lost in a world of crappy, nutritionally empty zombie foods disguised as seemingly healthy solutions.

Now the healthy food products that are minimally processed with quality ingredients are jumping on the bandwagon so people can easily identify the foods they want. Some of my items I get will have ten different icons on there, and I always get teased by my family, "What is it if it's free of pretty much everything else"? I have to chuckle too because all the marketing can just be too much to take at times. I still fall back to reading ingredients, always.

As I explained when giving up gluten, I instantly experienced positive results with my health. Of course, I didn't want to feel crappy again so it was much easier to make different food choices.

At first, this didn't eliminate fast food for me. I'd just get bun-less burgers, but because it was just such a pain in the ass to eat that way, I began eating a bit more at home which required some cooking and often included healthy, whole foods. The majority of the gluten foods I consumed were processed foods, so my taste for processed foods began to change as well.

I'd say during the remainder of the year that I was continually disappointed with the taste of fast food as I swear it was as though someone was switching out all the food for something else and it no longer tasted good to me. Today, there's only one restaurant I will eat at that could be kind of related to fast food, but it doesn't have a drive-thru if that tells you anything.

Because this was such a clear cause and effect for me, I slowly began eating more whole foods instead of zombie foods and my tastes for different foods began to change. I was bringing my taste buds out of their over salted-sugared-processed food coma with real food, and my body was telling me, "More, more, more." This is how your cravings can work for you instead of against you.

All of the foods that had gluten in it in my diet were very processed foods. I know for a fact that part of the amazing results with going gluten-free had much to do with giving up all of these foods. By default, in doing so, I began consuming more whole foods which also provided me the nutrition I'd been missing. But the process didn't happen overnight. I didn't cut gluten and start eating a ton of vegetables every day. It was a slow progression.

I have tried homemade bread from our local farmer's market that is wheat based. Regretfully, it doesn't taste nearly as good as it smells, and it still made my head dizzy, even with a small bite.

I basically did a smaller scale elimination diet and this set the course for me to be able to continually reduce the intake of foods that were not agreeing with me. An elimination diet, if you want to see about getting a clear connection of cause and effect with food, may be a good trial for you. There are many current plans out there that promote this, or you can do it on your own simply by eliminating some of the major processed foods you eat.

Two things happen when you do this. One, you eliminate empty calories and you consume nutritionally dense foods. Two, you get the nutrition you've been missing and you give your body a break from unhealthy foods. Excellent.

The idea being that, eventually, you introduce different foods back into your diet to see how you feel. Some people notice a clear change right away while others won't notice until after trying foods again how it impacts them or if it does at all. Aim for healthy food choices and minimally processed choices when you do introduce different foods back into your routine.

If you find this idea to be overwhelming, you don't have to drop everything at once, you can do this at your own pace and in your own way. You don't have to go from living off of fast food to gourmet cooking overnight. Rather, if your favorite meal is a burger and fries, make it at home instead of going out to eat. Little steps at a time will help a lot.

You may first just start by cutting back on sugar from either all the foods you eat or from sweets or both. You may work on adding in healthier foods, which is how you can begin to acquire a taste for fruits and vegetables, as I mentioned before.

What you can start doing to determine what processed foods are good for you and which foods are bad for you is simple. Instead of reading the nutrition panel to break down the calories, fat, sugar, salt, and percentages of each item, read the ingredients. Then, go to your trusty internet search engine friend and search like you're creepin' on your ex's Facebook page (I know you never do that), and find out what these ingredients are. I cannot, of course, vouch for the credibility of all information you will find, but I'm sure you're smart enough to figure it out. If you'd like to learn more about this, you can look at the resource guide for more information.

When you get overwhelmed by this information, remember to take a breather and walk away. It can be a bit daunting, and let's face it, sensationalism is used a lot these days and much of this information, though it is very important, can be explained in rather frightening manners. I mean, I guess I don't know how else it should be explained, but remember to take it all one step at a time.

I remember when I first learned about high-fructose corn syrup and hydrogenated oils on the *Dr. Oz* show and was totally panicked. In fact, it was years before I ever actually made changes based on what I learned watching his program.

Rest assured, you can do amazing things by making changes now to your lifestyle. I grew up on processed food also, many of us did, but the body is amazing, and with the food, love, and self-care you can provide, amazing healing can take place both mentally and physically.

Some of the overwhelming feelings clients of mine get are feelings of helplessness, not being able to make any changes, especially when realizing there are more zombie foods on the shelves in our homes, restaurants, and schools. Remember, you do have the ability to make a difference. It is already beginning with more and more food products available that are free from artificial ingredients, chemicals, and colors. Continue to be an informed consumer and shop accordingly. Your pocketbook makes all the difference. Where your dollars go will create demand for new and different food products and options.

Thankfully, now, since I'm eating whole foods and healthy food products, I find that I know when I'm full, but I don't know how to describe what I feel physically because I usually do not feel stuffed or heavy or bloated like I used to. It is more of an intuition or just knowing I'm done. I maintain my weight easily and don't feel the need to overdo it on certain types of foods. I still have the "treat" items I enjoy, but it's on a much smaller scale now than before, and though I may crave certain foods or desserts, it's no longer an uncontrollable force. It's more of a little thought that easily gets turned off with the day's events.

My diet is not perfect, but it continually improves. Yes, I still go out to eat and some places would be considered fast food. But I'm okay with that because, overall, I know I'm doing well with taking care of myself, not just with food, but in my life as well.

— eleven —

Burn Your Food and Be Happy

Most of us know that if you want to eat healthy you have to cook. Let's face it, with work, traffic, chores, bills, kids, dates, happy hours, TV shows, stress, and an utter lack of talent in the kitchen, cooking can be a real pain–I get it. I used to hate cooking. Some days, I still don't want to cook and I'm fine taking a night off, but it's nothing like I used to be. On most days, I cook all three of my meals, and I don't do a lot of prep. Mostly because I'm a creature of habit and eat the same stuff over and over again. Some see this as a flaw. I see this as a convenience to not have to do as much meal planning. Work with what you got, girl.

First and foremost, your home cooked meals do not have to be award winning beautiful meals, especially when you're just starting out. You know, the Pinterest gone wrong photos? Aim for that when trying a new recipe, not because I think all of you will be awful, but because it takes the pressure off, makes you laugh, and can make the experience, well, maybe even fun. You will overcook or steam your veggies and have them be all mushy. You will burn your food, and it'll be okay.

One night, while eating dinner with my husband, I had a case of the overly mushy vegetables. I ate most of my main part, probably chicken or a burger or something, but the half plate of overcooked zucchini, onions, and peppers was just not doing it for me. I said to him, "I'm still hungry." He says,

"Well, eat your vegetables. You have half your plate there."

Childhood rage boiled inside of me as invisible laser beams of temper tantrum filled rage met his gaze. "Do. Not. Tell. Me. To. Eat. My. Vegetables." The look must have been enough alone to get the point across because he looked a little frightened.

"I'm an adult, I buy my food too, and if I don't like my own cooking, I can choose to eat something else, damn it." He was now waiving a white flag of surrender—anything to make the scary face go away.

I get it. There's nothing worse than cooking and spending all this time and effort in the kitchen only to have your meal turn out awful. Been there, done that. Will do it again.

How many times have you gone out to eat and had only a mediocre meal, be it healthy or not? It's just kind of eh, okay, or maybe downright awful. Do you stop going out to eat? Sure, you may not visit the same place again, but you still go out to restaurants. Well, then why expect after one bad cooking experience in your kitchen that you should never cook again? Give yourself a break.

Here are some things I have done personally on my ventures into the kitchen and have also done in the cooking classes I teach. I will tell you right now that I am not a star cook. I am average, maybe with some things a little more advanced, but I overcook my chicken all of the time. Yet I have cooking classes, why? Because it is still decent food and because it's easy, minimal ingredients and most of it revolves around throwing food in the oven.

Rule numero uno: Do not cook hungry, hangry, or any variation of the two. You will more than likely ruin your meal anyway and then be even more irritated. Snack before and/or during your cooking process. If you spoil your appetite, yay for leftovers! You probably won't though.

Rule numero dos: Cheat when trying new recipes. If the recipes calls for chopped up garlic cloves, buy the minced garlic or use garlic powder. Is it the same? Of course not, but it'll work and it'll save time and frazzled feelings of frustration when having to chop five other vegetables. If the recipes calls for four different kinds of dried spices, use one of those pre-made bottles of spices with a generic flavor on it like "Hamburger Heaven" or "Chicken Yowza" (Okay, so my names are a bit sillier, but you know what I mean). They're spices and flavor, and ultimately, that's your goal, right? To make food with flavor?

Rule numero tres: Relax. Have a glass of wine, beer, coffee, water, milkshake. Whatever will make you feel relaxed, turn on some music, put on comfortable clothes. Don't fret and rush and feel as though everything has to be done, now, now, now. Also, keep in mind how long it takes to go out to eat– yes, it is easier in that you get to sit and unwind, but it takes time. If you give yourself the full amount of time it'd take to get to the restaurant, wait for your table, place your order, eat, pay, and drive home, would that be an hour? Would it be more or less? Well, then give yourself the same time and the same *type* of time. Go sit down for a few minutes. Change clothes. Unplug. Don't just jump right in the kitchen. Time yourself, too, from the start of cooking to the end of the meal. See how long it actually takes, and remember, each time you do this, it'll get better in the time it does take.

Rule numero cuatro: Be realistic about your expectations, skill level, and results. Don't plan to cook every night if you hardly cook at all. Start small first. Don't start with complicated recipes. Start with pre-made items so you can get the basics down pat.

Rule numero cinco: Have a backup plan for those unfortunate kitchen mishaps. We all have them. You boil hemp hearts thinking it is quinoa (that was my husband, not me). You forget to set the timer on the oven or what not. Have frozen foods, cereal, and a convenient takeout place on hand—something or anything so you can write it off and move on.

Rule numero seis: Make it social. If you have a family, get them involved and turn it into a game. If you are on your own, have dinner or brunch parties or dessert parties. Do potlucks or attend cooking classes. Host a YouTube cooking party and have friends over and everyone can try a different cooking technique via YouTube.

Rule numero something: Don't niche yourself into the same old techniques. Grill, use a wok, blend stuff, and be curious, just try things to try them. I'll take those bagged veggies that are made up for coleslaw and dump them in with my stir fry. They are vegetables, why not?

Some other basic tips: If you're a beginner, then pick a main dish OR a side item to make and purchase a pre-made something for the rest of the meal. Say, pick up a rotisserie chicken but you roast some veggies or make a great salad. Or you roast your own chicken breasts or fish and pick up sides of coleslaw or salad at your grocery store.

The key to remember here is it doesn't have to be perfect, you're not going to cook all of the time, and you can and will get better and more comfortable in the kitchen.

Also, make meals you are actually excited to eat. I can't tell you how many times I have clients talk about salads for eating healthy. Salad or plain chicken breast. It is exhausting. Listen, people don't want to live a plain chicken life. We want flavor and taste and excitement, so pick some meals you *want* to eat and you'll likely want to cook more. It may not start out as the healthiest meal, but give it time.

When making a healthy meal that is new for you, if the entire meal isn't something you're excited about or maybe a little nervous about trying, add a treat to it as a dessert or a side dish.

Try different ethnic styles of cooking and foods. You will likely find new ways to cook and new flavors. Look up vegetarian or vegan recipes just to try. There are some amazing ways to prepare vegetables that come out really fabulous, and it's a great way to have a healthy dish.

Go out to eat somewhere different, order veggies that you normally don't eat just to see how they taste and how they are prepared. If you don't like it, no harm, no foul. Experience food and cooking for what it is—something that can be fun, healthy, and a chance to explore food in your own way.

When you cook and buy more produce, you make new friends. Really, it's true. I know I did. Late one Saturday night, my husband and I were getting groceries–party! I was stocking up on produce and went to load up on Brussel sprouts when I noticed something odd looking stacked in the pile of little green cabbages. Looked like a rock.

Getting closer to the sprout, the supposed rock moved and out popped two little antennae, and a slimey, curious little snail. Excitedly, I picked up the large sprout he'd taken residence on and sneakily went to find my husband. I kept the sprout-surfing-snail under hand cover until I got to my husband who looked at me oddly while I ran up to him, gleefully smiling.

I remember him shaking his head saying, "Only you would find a critter at the grocery store. Go give him to an employee." "Oh, heck no! They'd just kill him or throw him out in the cold winter night," to which he replied, "Well, what are you going to do, carry him through the entire store?" So, I did what any logical person would do, I stole the Brussel sprout, rescued the snail, and made a break for the car. This new friend just got me out of grocery duty. We made it to the pet store before they closed and got a little set-up for him. The pet store worker was definitely jealous of my little new friend, who I named Goober.

Now, every time I get Brussel sprouts, I look for yet another snail. I figure if I find another snail, I better start playing the lotto because who has that happen twice, right? But most times I'm at the grocery store, it's just plain old shopping time. Though there are instances when I look down at my shopping cart and think, "Wow, look at how healthy this is. Who's going to eat all these veggies?"

Lasting change takes time to build and it seemed as though some changes I implemented, at times, were just silly because they were so *small*, but these small changes added up to lasting habits. Your journey to a healthier lifestyle will usually not have an end or a final point.

What you will experience is the confidence to be able to feel more like yourself AND not feel dominated by the stress of eating the "right" foods or overdoing it on the "wrong" foods.

I still enjoy my treat type food items and I don't stress about it as I used to stress – pizza, fries, or a baked good or sweet item still has its place in my life, and now, when I have a craving for some of these foods, I can easily think through whether or not I really want to have it or if it is the idea of picking up a pizza and not cooking. If so, I ask myself, "What else is easy?"

twelve

Health Is More than Weight

A few years ago, this great friend of mine kept telling me to go see her doctor. She swore by his methods and that he could help me with everything I had problems with. That was a tall order and I certainly had my doubts.

Anyway, I put her off for months because I was a crabby skeptic and wanted to keep trying all the same methods that had failed me many times. Then I got what felt like an awful UTI and I went to a specialist to get it checked out. This was not my first rodeo at all, as I mentioned, I was very familiar with problems concerning the lady parts. It began in my teenage years and it happened a lot—feeling like I had a UTI yet when I'd go get checked out, nothing showed up. I mean, heck, I drank water only, rare for a teenager to not have some kind of sugary beverage, but I never really liked soda, so that was a plus in my favor.

And this particular instance was no exception to my past experiences. I went in to see a urologist who did a bladder catheter–OUCH! And other tests. As if getting a catheter isn't pleasant enough, the doctor wanted to give me the 101 of vaginal care, as though I hadn't been caring for my lady parts for the twenty plus years I'd been alive. She offered her first line in the speech before I took over:

"I don't drink sugary beverages. I drink lots of water. I

wash with mild or no soap and warm water. I don't wear overly tight clothing. I don't stay in wet or damp clothes. (Who does that, really?) I'm aware of the potential irritation from shaving or douching and all of the pros and cons and warnings of each."

You'd think I just told a kid Santa isn't real with the look on her face. She had nothing else to tell me. I knew and heard it all. Like I said, not my first rodeo.

After the very uncomfortable test was completed and the initial urine results were back, the report I was given was, "Your urine is unremarkable." At this, I knew the look I had on my face, "What exactly are you saying here, doc?" While the crickets chirped and I waited for the follow-up, I got the sneaking feeling I knew nothing was going to be solved today.

That was correct. There was absolutely no sign or indication that there was anything in there even remotely close to an infection. Of course, it was because I drink water like a camel.

I was prescribed antibiotics anyway and out of pain and desperation, I took them.

A few days later, and after rounds of diarrhea, I called the nurse and explained my experience. Not only was the pain not gone, but now I was having embarrassing and uncomfortable bowel activity. I was told that's not a side effect and to continue treatment.

I begged to differ. Seeing as how that was the only change to my routine, I went ahead and stopped taking them and made a call I'd been meaning to get to for weeks.

My dear friend's doctor finally became a priority for me, so I called him and thankfully, he had a cancellation the next day so I was able to get in quickly.

At my appointment, I explained my full laundry list of problems I was currently or have regularly dealt with—UTI like symptoms with no sign of infection, acne, lack of energy, dermatitis, anxiety, headaches, shoulder and neck pain, acid reflux, phlegm and drainage in my throat, and, oh, I ride the emotional rollercoaster regularly.

He poked and prodded, literally, and did a lot of random stuff, none of which was nearly as uncomfortable as previous appointments, but also not like anything I'd ever experienced. Upon arriving at his office, I learned he practices chiropractic and applied kinesiology, two new experiences for me, aside from a few other chiropractors here and there over the years.

At the end of the appointment, I asked about what he can do for my urinary tract symptoms and pain since it didn't seem we had covered that at all yet. He told me he was going to send me home with something to take that should alleviate the pain. I left irritated and with some sticker shock at the price of the appointment and the herbal supplement. I felt as though I had no answers or solutions, and less money.

Being the ever good patient, I got home that night and drank half of the suggested amount of the supplement he provided me with. Not because I didn't want to take it all, I just didn't have the right size measuring spoon so I guessed. I learned later I was taking half the dosage.

After a couple swigs down, by the next morning, much to my

surprise, my pain was greatly reduced. It went from a *"leave me the hell alone"* to *"Hey, how you doing?"* (Complete with head nod and all.)

No blazing flames of glory this morning. My pain was reduced to at least half the level it'd been previously. I continued drinking the supplement and within a couple of days, I felt much better with no symptoms. After this experience, unbeknownst to him, he became the solution to my problems. Poor schmuck.

Three or so years have passed and he has been instrumental in helping me implement changes to feel better, eat better, and kick bad food cravings right out the window. Oh, and since I have no filter at my appointments (after you tell someone about your urinary tract pain, there's not many topics that'll leave you shy), he kind of doubles as my bartender or shrink because I unload my personal problems on him as well. Of course, he just laughs at me and reminds me, "That's called baggage." One time, he even did a little dance and sang out, "That's called baggage," while lifting his imaginary suitcases.

In my time working with him, I have come a long way and have learned when making changes to your mental, emotional, and physical health, having support is key. So regardless of *what* path you choose for support, follow what works for you. There are all kinds of practitioners out there and they all have their place, time, and expertise. Sure, I've had some rough experiences in the traditional world of medicine, but I have had some really great experiences and physicians as well. I just had to keep exploring my options.

Support can come in all manner of speaking. Since I am

sharing my experience with improving my health with you, I can't overlook my primary food areas, which are also something that required a lot of TLC.

With respect to primary foods, I had a lot to focus on because I wanted to meet someone and I had no professional direction, which were the two most demanding deficiencies I dealt with. I worked whatever job I could settle for, assuming it was still the way of the world to work for security, benefits, and money only without actually *also* getting to enjoy one's work, or better yet, fulfill your purpose.

I figured, sometime down the line, I'd surely get a job and like it and that would be that. I'd be like someone out of a movie with the fancy office and nice clothes and all is well with the world. Boy, did I have a lot to learn, starting with figuring out what the heck I wanted to do with the rest of my life.

Eventually, I went back to college to get my degree in communications after having read *Life 101: Everything We Wish We Had Learned about Life in School–But Didn't* by Peter McWilliams. It was the first exposure I had to self-help and I was hooked. I wanted to write a book, I didn't know what about or how, but I knew it'd be about a lot of great stuff and about not being bad for being emotional–long standing soapbox there.

Still, after getting my degree, I couldn't find a job I liked nor did I really have a clear idea of what I wanted to do. Sure, there were a few thoughts here or there, but nothing that was really driving me to what felt like the way to go. That was until I found the Institute for Integrative Nutrition a year after graduating college. I enrolled within a few weeks. (My husband always said I have one speed: full steam ahead. I knew that was true with our relationship, but I didn't think it was in other areas of my life. Yet, when I heard about the adult program at the college I attended, I was enrolled within a few weeks, same with IIN, enrolled in a few weeks. But as I tell him with having met him, when you got a good thing, you don't wait around or let it go.)

I knew I was onto something good. I knew I was finally tapping into something I felt passionate about and was going to enjoy doing. Since then, it's been an up and down exciting ride of figuring out what to do next and having a lot of great chances to learn and grow.

I've made many mistakes along the way, and I know I still will, but learning and moving forward is so important. I have had help and support from my friends and family and have had to learn to be there for myself.

All of these primary food deficiencies were already in the works before I found the support I needed with my health and wellness, and I continue to nourish each area of my life as days pass.

I really love the word "nourish." It feels like a warm sweater and a crisp pair of jeans on a brisk, sunny autumn day. I can really settle into this word. Nourishment can come in the form of foods you eat to how you are living your life and spending your time, which we will look into further in the primary foods chapter. Nourishment will be different for everyone and will continually change throughout your lifetime.

The weight loss industry is on the over-advertised, thin quick side, and doesn't put a lot of focus on health or eating for your health. It is assumed that if you lose weight then you are becoming healthier. Yet, we all know of some crazy practices people may follow in order to see weight loss results that are certainly not healthy.

Providing nourishment to your mind, body, and spirit through primary foods, secondary foods, and tapping into yourself is an entirely different experience than dieting for weight goals. It is going to be different for each person, and the complex and deep levels of accepting yourself and your ability and your right to walk your own path, call your own shots, and shake it up will be empowering, enlightening, and well, challenging, but in all the right ways.

Yes, you want to lose weight. I understand. I've been there. I've yo-yoed thirty-five pounds on and off over the years, I've been heavier than I wanted, and I've been under weight. But by focusing on your health, you will not only be able to more easily obtain and manage your desired weight, you will also alleviate various physical symptoms through nourishment and healing. Unfortunately, many of the healing dietary theories available get lumped into one big industry of weight loss and may get a bad rap when that's often not the case.

Today, we are dealing with the fallout from processed foods dominating our daily food intake. We are dealing with a whole host of problems we've not yet encountered. Many of the healing plans today are created with this in mind. We have to heal the problems that come from ingesting processed foods and also build up the nutrition we have been missing from a lack of local, seasonal, fresh, or whole foods.

We have become accustomed to vegetables being on our sandwich toppings, in a salad, or as a side dish. Vegetables are no side dish. They should be the main star of the show.

Because of this unique situation, there are people who are seeking solutions for other health concerns aside from weight loss and that is why so many different theories are now present, which are based on bio-individual needs.

I am gluten-free and dairy-free most of the time with the occasional pizza or use of butter when cooking. I mentioned how after going gluten-free, I kind of fell into a paleo way of eating and that continues to change as I continue to take care of my health. A while back, I began following the Anti-Candida Diet because I was battling an overgrowth of Candida in my gut. It was a pretty strict protocol. I was hoping to alleviate many symptoms I've had like anxiety, dermatitis, cold hands and feet (I always stick my cold feet under or near my husband and give him a good goose, which is fun), mood swings, and a constant craving for sugar.

I was really fed up with feeling anxious and worried about *everything* all of the time. Not just a little worry—it was jumping to worst case scenarios always and being on edge over it. I definitely noticed a connection with certain foods impacting my worries and anxiety and concerning imagination. So when I had a chance to reduce or eliminate this pain in my life, I jumped on it. I got on the Anti-Candida Diet, which for those unfamiliar with it, means I couldn't have *any* sugar, even fruit, at least to start.

I stuck with it for a long time, and I did the most intense version of it, longer than what was necessary. Not having any sugar causes the Candida fungus to starve and die.

I remember researching Candida and finding numerous bloggers sharing how they beat it, and each one had a different something they did that seemed to help.

Once again, as with the way my schooling went, contradicting information was a plenty. One person had success, but didn't have to cut out this type of food, while another didn't have any success on this diet, but followed GAPS, Gut and Psychology Syndrome protocol, instead, while another had a lot more success going paleo or using the Body Ecology Diet. The list went on and on.

This is exactly why bio-individuality is such a key point to remember, so I began tapping back in and trusting myself to make changes and select the food I knew to be healthy for me, and to continue to steer clear of unhealthy foods *for me*. Instead, I began to read about each of these different protocols and cherry picking different tips from each plan. It wasn't easy, and as I mentioned, I overdid it with the most intense version of the Anti-Candida Diet for too long because I was so hopeful to see improvements, and in many ways, I did, but not entirely. I also began stressing myself out too much about every little thing I could or couldn't eat.

What I started to see, however, was a clear pattern in all the dietary theories I found that helped many of the issues I was dealing with. Usually, all of the vegetables and proteins were the same—high fermented foods, high plant foods, and low sugary and starchy foods, no processed foods. Before I'd even really heard of half of these diets, even from school, I was naturally pulling in these foods either from personal taste or just because I could tell they were better choices based on how I was feeling.

Most of us want some answers, guidance, or sanity in this process and I will tell you that there are some great healing plans out there that will support not only weight loss, but most importantly, your health. But I don't believe it's that easy. I think of ebb and flow of learning, taking one step at a time based on finding something that sounds feasible, sensible to you, and then apply what does work for you and don't force the aspects that do not suit your needs.

For instance, after realizing being gluten-free was a great change for me and learning paleo recipes would be good gluten-free options, I knew if I wanted to get a recipe for a meal or baked good, I could find paleo recipes and be in good shape because I know their recipes include foods that are healthy *for me.*

As I became exposed to additional theories, what I found interesting was that the Anti-Candida Diet, Body Ecology Diet, and the GAPS Diet were all inclusive of foods I was already eating on a regular basis and consisted mostly of the vegetables I prefer to eat. What I then began doing was cherry picking the most bang for my buck recommendations from each of these plans.

For instance, the Body Ecology Diet discusses combining foods in a manner to support digestion, and eating fermented foods which are naturally rich in probiotic—bacteria we need to support a healthy gut, immune system, and digestion. These practices made sense to me so I figured instead of doing a huge overhaul, I'm going to practice these two and see what happens.

There are many dietary theories or plans that may provide great benefit to you, but don't be afraid to use these protocols in your own manner because you will feel and experience the results first hand. And if you then decide it is worth exploring further, go for it. Everyone will have different levels of what will be useful and beneficial, and some of you may find that various healing plans aren't so hard once you get healthy results and you can integrate them more and more into your daily routine. It may feel more easy and natural for you to do.

The proof is in the pudding, friends. We have all seen someone go through these kinds of amazing transformations from people who find a way to improve their health and are seemingly like a different person, right? And we all want to know is their story–*their* story and individual experience. Now it is time to read your past story and begin listening to *your* inner narrator, inner wisdom, inner eager student, whatever you want to call that side of yourself. When you tap into the changes that suit you, you'll know by all the amazing experiences that you will begin to have much more than weight loss.

thirteen

What Are You *Able* to Do?

I see in our society and in the industry I'm working in a lot of various forms of pressure to either eating the "right" way or the "wrong" way, and everyone could be doing it wrong or right, depending on whom you ask.

I've been this person long before I went through my training to become a health coach, and I've heard it from others in and out of the industry. It's all on the individual and we get really miffed when others aren't doing what they *should* be doing. Bear with me on this rant because it really does tie in to your daily treatment of yourself.

Remember the anger discussion, the energy for change? It is overly misused either on empty matters that don't require *your* energy for change (other people's business) or by silly matters like traffic, crappy television shows, or a messed up order from a restaurant.

But anger is also often rewarded. We all love that "go off on you" segment in the movies when it's something good or someone is seemingly deserving of it. Combine that with our need to "fix" everything and we can absolutely lose sight of how to use anger to our benefit, and it becomes to our detriment.

Say, for instance, you are dealing with someone in a scenario where they seem as though they are making excuses as to why they can't do this or that. Do you get miffed or irritated? Do you find yourself thinking, "Well, it is your own fault. Why don't you do something about it?"

Maybe they are being irresponsible, or maybe they messed up, or maybe they are just having a really horrible time unbeknownst to you and everyone around. If we just blame and shut them down, we are never going to learn and grow.

It is *easy* to blame people and dismiss the problem as, "Well, it's your own fault." That is not holding someone accountable, lacks empathy, understanding, or support, and replaces it with anger, judgment, or skeptic criticism. This is not what unconditional or tough love is about. It is about being there to support your person in the role you are—spouse, sister, friend, whoever.

I've done this. I've tried it this way and it doesn't work. You have to find a way to not judge, which is extremely challenging, and also to not take it personally when people may lash out at you and be angry with you for pointing out what they don't want to hear, or for not being able to fix their problems by your standards and by your time table.

It's also waaay easier for the one who is passing judgment to dismiss someone else's problems as being self-inflicted because then there's nothing you have to do about it to support or help this person. You don't have to be in the uncomfortable role of, "I want to help her, but how? What do I say, what do I do?" Or, "Geez, I'm so sick of hearing about these issues."

As a health coach, it's my job to think about things beyond what I know and not assume that everyone is a lazy bum or someone who just can't get their act together. It is really hard to accept people may actually just be having trouble putting one foot in front of the other. Though I don't understand it, it is real for them. This is not about bending rules for people or making exceptions—that's not what having empathy or being supportive is about. It's hearing them and being able to respect where they are at.

Pressure leads us to feel more desperate to be successful by not only our own means but by others' as well, and often times, our own success is compromised to make sure others are also pleased. I hear a lot about willpower and accountability in my line of work. Both, when understood and used properly, are key pieces of learning and reaching goals. When misunderstood and used ineffectually, are a paralysis to any lasting results with temporary boughs of progress here and there.

Account-*able* and response-*able* (yes, I am well aware of the typo, bear with me for the point of this matter) mean you have to be *able* to take action. A person has to have trust in themselves to be *able* to be held accountable for their actions and to respond to the different steps in each part of the process of weight loss and healthy lifestyle changes. If a person feels *unable* to do these things, then there is going to be a lot of hang up in even getting the process going.

This can be influenced by many factors, many internal and many external influential factors from the way others treat you, the experiences you have in life, and its impact on your self-esteem. We're like a little pinball getting bounced around by all these external influences in life, like someone who has that vibe of, "Gosh, you're so irresponsible." That means I'm holding you accountable, but I'm not really. I'm judging you because you're inconveniencing my day, because I don't like what you're doing and I can't "fix" you. I can't solve your problems.

From a social perspective, we like simple categories, labels, and solutions. Fix a problem. Here's some simple sentiment that will "fix" you. Done. Sometimes, small problems can fit in a neat category and be handled in a textbook manner and life is great.

People have many layers and many feelings, and there are usually many solutions to a problem that need to be explored. We forget that we need to be present with a person instead of trying to "fix" them. Sometimes, the best help we have is just being *there*.

I've learned this the painful way by not being a good support for people who are close to me, and by also missing the support I needed for myself from others. We've all made big mistakes like this or had to learn the hard way. I am still working on it. It's easy to fall into this routine, especially when dealing with those you care most about because of the helpless feelings building into anger.

Holding yourself or others accountable is not about punishment, guilt, anger, feelings of inadequacy, or shame. It's about recognizing your ability to do something, and as hard as it may be to trust yourself, to be *able* to do something, you've got to start somewhere and then be able to trust yourself to take one step in the direction *you* want to go.

If you keep trying something, you are reinforcing, "I am *able* to do something, and decide yes, I want to eat healthy," and then put forth the steps needed to keep trying different things. Take action, and turn actions into accomplishments.

Being account-able means you are able to account for your actions. Sometimes it may sound like a bunch of BS excuses. "I started my workouts and then my kid got sick, my schedule changed, I got dumped." Basically, there was a plan and something threw it off track. "I don't have any willpower to stick to a diet," or, "I was stressed or tired."

You are holding yourself accountable in this stream of what we recognize as simple BS excuses. You are an adult and you are still learning, and it is okay if it takes you fifty freaking times to learn and get a new routine going. It is okay that you have to figure out through trial and error how to make changes because you are likely working against habits that have been in place for a long time, and you have to restructure your habits while also dealing with day-to-day demands that are depleting your energy and willpower without always having ways to replenish your energy and willpower.

We don't give ourselves a break enough. There's a lot of focus on exhausting ourselves to work hard, earn more money, get that promotion, buy that new whatsadoodle. It's part of the norm to be hard on ourselves. But then the problems are never being dealt with, the root cause of poor lifestyle choices are not being taken into consideration, and we are not holding ourselves accountable to *all* of the healthy lifestyle changes we need to implement.

Get back to those primary food imbalances and deficiencies

and hold yourself accountable to making improvements there. There is this complex array of all these things going on. When you get stuck, I want you to think, "What are you *able* to do?" You are able to *respond* to what is going on, these excuses you have. What *can* you do to start changing these scenarios? I want you to think, "I am able," when you get mad and feel stuck.

When you begin to think more about what you are *able* to do, you may find you begin to stop carrying that which you don't like, and you'll free up all this energy to *do* other things, even if it's the little stuff. Pay attention to how much more you make comments like, "I hate that song," or, "I hate this kind of weather," or, "I don't like the smell of...," so on and so forth. Replace these with indifferent thoughts of acknowledgement and then let them go. For this, I highly recommend additional mental exercises such as guided meditation or visualization. You don't have to like everything, but it doesn't need to take your energy to dislike it.

We are very creative beings. We are meant to be moving, and doing, and creating, and challenged, both mentally and physically. Now, many of us sit on our ass, only being mentally challenged, but not physically, and sometimes, not mentally stimulated in the ways in which we crave. After draining our mental power and then not using the physical energy you have, motivation begins to dissipate. "Oh, guess I'm not needed here. I'll go elsewhere then." Leaving you at the end of your day, sitting on your ass, feeling exhausted. It becomes really hard to gain or spark some kind of energy at the end of your work day to get to the gym or cook dinner.

The common workweek in our culture is Monday through

Friday, workin' nine to five, and by the time you get home, there's no umph left in your day to do all the things you want to do before it's time for bed, preparing to do it again tomorrow.

For those who are physically taxed at their job, they may be ready to wind down physically, but their minds may still be active or busy.

We are so removed from the outdoors and we don't have nearly as many physical demands to take care of in our day-to-day lives, we are trying to find ways to get that creative spark to get us fired up or to "do" something. So then it becomes a need we need to satisfy and this may be fulfilled by empty means—junk food, alcohol, drugs, sex, television, shopping, or drama and conflict.

All of these things can provide both quality satisfaction or empty satisfaction, depending on how, when, why, who, it's engaged, but much of it in today's culture is over used, abused, and taken for granted, or used to mask what feels impossible to fix due to social expectations both internally and externally.

We often feel entitled to tell one another when we are going to make a mistake because we're on the outside looking in. This undermines other's ability to trust and hear their inner wisdom–we are actually mirroring our own insecurities and doubts and set ourselves up to need and seek approval of others in fear of making mistakes. "Will I screw up if I make this career change?" "Will I not get another date if I text too soon?" It undermines our own *ability* to make decisions, deal with whatever results we may get, and to move on having learned from a situation.

(If you haven't caught the broken record message of learning yet, it'll keep coming at ya. And for those who may be out there braving the dating game, it doesn't matter when you text someone or how open you are to sharing your feelings. Either they're the right person or not. They'll either be charmed by your overexcited texting and have the same feelings back, or they'll be turned off by it, but if you're curbing your behavior from the get-go trying to be someone else, then it'll not last anyway. Hang in there.)

We then undermine our own ability to make decisions. It's always easy to say *you're* making a mistake because you aren't me and you aren't walking in my shoes. In our advice seeking, it gets so jumbled up with opinions from this person and that person and they are all going to be different, and more than likely, you're going to follow the person who mirrors the same thoughts you initially felt and doubted in the first place when really, all you needed was some validation and support from someone who cares about you.

The spark to advise, fix, or help others can be a positive aspect in our day-to-day lives, but sometimes it gets fueled by anger. After a while, anger becomes consuming energy, and it may make you feel amped up, but it usually it becomes hard to let go because you then need to find something else to do and another source of energy.

I used to seek out shows that provided that conflict for me to get that little outlet for conflict or drama, and granted, I make good choices about what shows I watch, and it's better to watch drama that is perfectly resolved in a few minutes as opposed to creating drama in my day-to-day life with the people around me.

What if instead of putting energy out there to change everything around us, we began focusing that energy on what we don't take in when being in a situation, looking around, and trying to ignore being irritated or angry? What is going on that is positive that is around you right now? What are these dislikes taking away from? What do I miss as a coach if I only get angry and take it personally every time a client comes to me with failed attempts, or with resistance to my coaching?

What am I missing? Because I'm carrying all of this anger that's taking my time, energy, and focus. Like a kid's bad behavior, we get so wrapped up in their unwanted behavior (and for good reason when we're fearful of the outcome and their wellbeing), that we sometimes forget to stop and ask, "How are you doing?" Or say, "Let's just hang out and shoot the bull and just talk or go do something fun."

What are you hurting from, or is there something you're scared of? What is the real problem at hand, and how can we look at the good and use this instead of trying to control the bad behavior? Also, vulnerability and sadness are important indicators as well.

Then it comes to responsibility and whether or not everyone is being responsible, and in order to do that, I have to control and punish because that's what holds people accountable and teaches them cause and effect. Cause and effect really happens all on its own.

Control gets inspired by fear. I'm a half-assed doomsday prepper because of my own worries and fears around the need to plan for and control different scenarios.

I stock piled totally random stuff in my car as I headed out the door, like saving a half-eaten granola bar in my car. Or I'd pile up random clothing items to keep in the car during winter time, never really knowing what I did and didn't have.

It was all because I wanted to feel prepared and *able* to handle and control every situation that could potentially happen and scare me. But in my haste and fear, I didn't really invest in a productive and realistic plan, nor did I accept that life is messy and we are going to experience challenges and events that can't be planned for or escaped, but they may be survived.

Control through anger and dominance or shutting down emotions and creating roadblocks is not what stimulates growth, learning, self-love or compassion for others. It stops it.

Inner wisdom is as unique as your fingerprint, which is why so many different stories of healing, growth, and success in many areas of life, not just our health, are present. But trusting yourself and your ability to *forgive* and still love yourself through failures and through success is part of the process in hearing and being one with your inner wisdom.

Walking away from traditional methods and negative approaches of guilt or blame based accountability will be empowering and really rewarding. You will stumble no matter if you walk your own path or others', but when walking your own path, you will stumble onto something great, for you. It doesn't have to be for everyone, it doesn't have to even make sense to anyone else. It's all for you.

Inner wisdom is going to be for your ears only and hearing it means letting go of the comfort zone and taking a walk outside of it. Redefine your success to understand your intention, the hard work worth doing that will bring you success in your own actions and failures. Let yourself off the hook and forgive past perceived failures and begin learning from it. Use your excuses to operate within what you can do and what you cannot do, and hone in on what's left to put the pieces together.

fourteen

My Flaws Don't Make You Better

Body image issues. Every. One. Has. Them. Sure, you may think you'd like to deal with another's body type, size, and related issues, but the pain doesn't just go away. Body image issues are directly related to how you feel about yourself. It is another opportunity for your insecurities to flourish. Be it only a small insecurity or a real gorilla on you back, it's a common concern for men and women of all walks of life.

Never undermine your own pain or someone else's when it comes to their insecurities, no matter what they're tied to. But why do we care so much about ourselves and why do we care so much about others? Why are we jealous and feel insecure by other's looks or by being overly concerned about their physical appearance not being good enough? And why do we only care about flaws or tearing one another down?

We are pressured way too much to have the "perfect" body. Images are all around us of large breasted, slender, tan, and impossibly beautiful women. We are supposed to be seductive, sexy, curvy, and soft, yet firm all in one perfect package while holding a greasy hamburger and going to town like its 1999. Right. (Personal pet peeve, those commercials. I want to know how many mouthfuls of hamburger were spat out with gusto in between takes.)

Just as we have food messages bombarding us all day long,

157

we are laced with explicit images of women's bodies. I mean, whoever buys that lingerie commercials are actually geared toward women must be seriously inebriated. Also, I have never had a man actually venture into a lingerie store to buy me something. They only *look* at the catalogues if they get the chance. Marketing fail.

We've got food everywhere, overly sexual imagery in entertainment and advertising, sit on our butts for work, and wonder why we are all so hard on ourselves and seeking some magic solution to all our insecurities wrapped up in a simple ten step program that'll be ours in just five simple installments!

Sure, we can all joke and say things like, "Ya, I don't miss a meal!" or, "Makes me feel like I actually have [insert desired body part here]." But in all seriousness, aside from offhanded sarcastic comments to deflect or diffuse the real pain here, most people really want to make the pain around these insecurities go away and not rely on it for a punchline as in a manner to "apologize" to others for not being good enough.

Most of us don't want to openly talk about or pay attention to insecurities, body related or otherwise. And somehow, I don't know how this has taken shape to arrive at where we are now, but we find certain physical attributes to be the standard for all, and if we are not at that specific standard, it's quite alright to poke fun about it, be it about ourselves or others.

It's not limited to weight. It's anything from size, skin tone, cup size, height, strength, the amount of cellulite one has, or for men, it's height, body hair, strength, and overall size with not being too big, but not too little. I don't know if it is a result of all the imagery we are exposed to in the movies, entertainment industry, magazines and advertisements, or if somehow, we all want a similar look and berate ourselves and others when it isn't achieved.

I've heard comments made about small busted women. I've heard them from small busted women, and I've said it myself about myself. I've felt the embarrassment trying to shop for bras and nearly all of them being too big no matter how many little A's are on the tag.

One day, I even heard a gal in the bra department whining to her boyfriend about her good friend who buys these big padded bras and wears tight clothing. She was mad her friend was a "faker." I, being a fellow insecure member of the little boob club didn't feel the need to go start a dramatic scene at the Kohl's department store, but I felt bad. I also made damn sure I wasn't spotted by Busty McGhee. I don't hold a grudge, or well, didn't hold it for too long. For whatever reason, this made her so mad, and I have no doubt it's mirroring her own actions and insecurities too, and the pain is making her cranky.

Then later, I realized something really important. Men don't care about padded bras! Men usually don't notice. If the bra comes off, men are happy, thankful, and excited that YOU'RE NAKED! So be insecure, be nervous, but don't let that stand in the way of enjoying an intimate or romantic moment with someone. Likely, they are worrying about their own insecurities too!

I remember one time, my brother with his wild colored hair

in high school, told me about some kid who was giving him a hard time about his hair. He asked him, "Why do you dye your hair like that?" My brother calmly replied, "Why do you care?" This was exactly what I wanted to ask this gal—why in the world she really cares enough to actually be *angry* that her friend is buying padded bras? Oh, the nerve!

The comments I have said myself or have had others say to me regarding my weight and bust size have ranged from being playfully called nasty names for being able to wear a form fitting outfit to being chided for not having any boobs, all of which can sting a little or a lot. I've had people point out when I get too thin or when I have put on pounds, to treating me poorly for having lost weight too fast. I've even been told by many that I can't relate to what it feels like to be insecure about my body since I've always been on the smaller side. Again, ouch.

I wonder sometimes, why it is we either pick out our own flaws or feel it's necessary to comment on someone else's as though it's our right to make the flaws we find in others the butt of a joke? Or why is it that we assume others' complaints or pain is not real because we aren't living it? (Ugly truth about me—I've been the one assuming others don't really have it that bad, or feel it is okay to not be empathetic to their struggles because I don't get it. I've learned this the hard way by dishing it out, but also by being on the receiving end of the dish–and it's no bowl of ice cream, I can promise you that!)

We all have real insecurities and challenges, so don't diminish anyone else's struggles because they're not real for you, and don't let anyone else diminish your struggles in the same way.

But most importantly, do not diminish your self-worth by hyper-focusing on your insecurities. You may be the only one who notices them.

Countless women I have spoken with, be it friends, family, fellow shoppers in a store, the nurse weighing me at a doctor's appointment, we all share some similar struggles with body image, either as a whole or certain parts of it. After all, we all are our own worst critics, right?

Also, what's with this puberty bit in health class? It's another thing that needs modification. "When you begin to develop, your body will change." Develop? What am I, a roll of thirty-five millimeter? (Google it, youngin's.) It seemed implied that when breasts develop, this means breasts of a certain size, as though in order to develop properly they have to get to a particular size. Imagine my utter disappointment when this never happened for me. I was still waiting well into my twenties.

Not only have I been on the receiving end of comments like, "You have no ass," I have also not regularly gotten what I'd deem a sincere compliment. It's more of a backhanded sucker punch with a Band-Aid. You know what these are like—you sport a nice outfit and instead of saying, "Wow, you look great," they say something like, "You bitch!" or, "You suck, I'm so jealous right now."

Thanks, I think. As if somehow these words don't actually sting simply because, in your mind, I'm free of any insecurity. This just adds guilt to a scenario because other people are angered or playfully jealous by my looking good. For the record, I'm not exactly flattered by this kind of sentiment.

I much prefer to tell people, "Hey, I really like your outfit," or, "Hey, that color looks awesome on you." This is the way I prefer to compliment others as well. Oh, I know, roll your eyes. I'm so sensitive. They are just playing! When did it become so hard to be truly happy for others without having to hide it in sarcasm or playful hatin'?

I consider myself an average person. I have acne, cellulite, weird vein business going on, small boobs, and a tendency to get food stuck in my teeth. For the love of food, it kills me how many times I'll be out with people and have food in my teeth and no one says ANYTHING. Sometimes it's berry smoothie bits which can be huge chunks–nothing. I'm starting to think my husband's eyesight is VERY bad.

I could ramble on all day about other little or big things, but you get the idea. Yet I've still had those backhanded compliments sent my way.

It makes me think, what about those women who are drop dead knockouts? The ones who DO fit the mold of stereotypical body image standards—what pressure do they feel and experience? What do people say to *them* when they look great? Could you honestly imagine what it must feel like for those gals or guys, who are the models or "hot" chics/dudes you know from work, college, or wherever? What must that feel like on a daily basis? A friend told me once that her therapist said some of the people who suffer the most with self-worth are some of the most attractive women you'd ever see.

I remember this one day at work when one of the reps from this company walked by my door and, my goodness, he looked like a walking Calvin Klein ad. I nearly fell out of my chair and then proceeded to buzz my friend's extension, asking why in the blazes she had never mentioned this fine light of sunshine before AND warned a gal about actually putting on a nice outfit instead of loafers, mismatched socks, and an overall comfortable yet bordering on old age office attire. Geez! Hey, these were in my single and lonely days. This was a big deal for me.

Anyway, it seems to be that being super good looking must be like having a super power. Have you ever thought about all the attention, wanted or not, and all the social pressure or unjustified expectations? You'd have other women sizing you up, automatically thinking you're a snob, or you'd have everything handed to you because of your looks, you know, all the cattiness in the movies, TV, and in real life that we gals have dished out or been on the receiving end of. That's not even scratching the surface of how men treat women or how really attractive men are treated. I tend to assume that super hot guys are players, arrogant, and totally untrustworthy. (Until I married one, that is!)

I don't know about you, but when I've met or been around those really attractive people, I can't even function like a normal person. I am so intimidated it's like the words that usually fall out of my mouth at rapid pace just evaporate into thin air. It doesn't matter if it's the same sex or opposite sex, I just feel like a goofy, goofball.

I find myself feeling totally awkward, not sure what to say or how to act, or wondering if I suddenly have smeared lipstick, food in my teeth, or a hole in my clothes. I instantly feel a fart coming on and silently hope and pray to the flatulence powers that be for it to be silent and not overly ripe!

Seriously though, put yourself in the other person's shoes, the super attractive person. Can you imagine what it must feel like to create such uncomfortableness in others just by your appearance? They know they are having awkward conversations, they see the fidgets and nerves, I'm sure.

I mean, sure, sometimes it may be flattering, but what about when it becomes a true hindrance to your daily interactions with others and the ability to develop more important relationships? Ever say, "He/She is so nice even though they are so attractive," or something along those lines? As if being so attractive instantly means they should be unfriendly or a mean person.

So I really think we always assume others have it easy, but everyone has something to battle, no matter how much better they seem to have it. We all have our own demons, struggles, and worries.

And fixing one won't fix everything, which I can speak from experience after having worked my hiney off before flying to Cancun and feeling really great about my physique, I still had plenty of other insecurities and doubts to get distracted by. Will I say something totally stupid when I talk? Did I already say something stupid? Is my dermatitis causing flakes in my hair to float around? What's that smell, is it me, did I put on deodorant? Do I have something in my teeth?

Women aren't the only one who deal with this pressure. We often think men have it easier. And in some cases, maybe. But I think men have a different problem. They have to be tough, strong, and often big. Many times, we don't care what kind of big, just big. Broad shoulder, solid, strong legs, muscular, etc.

If a woman says she is on a diet, some of her friends may chime in on how great she looks and that she doesn't need to diet, and of course, encourage her to eat, which that isn't really a good thing, but well intended. Men, however, often don't openly say, "I'm on a diet," because of the way he may look to his peers, especially the men who need it most—the bigger the guy, the more he is expected to eat, drink, and scratch. Er, well, maybe not that last part, but you get the idea.

Really, male stereotypical expectations are awful. They aren't supposed to show much emotion, they need to be able to provide, fix stuff, and do man things, whatever that may entail. Males who are too soft or sensitive are less manly. Men who are too smart are not bad boy enough. Men are stupid or all men are hornballs. This gets played out to an exhausting level and I've seen it with respect to how they take care of their own health, as in they don't.

It ain't a problem unless it's bleeding and falling off. So a man who is the big guy and automatically supposed to be tough is also supposed to polish off gobs of junk food, not eat a lot of sissy food or health foods, and drink a lot to boot.

But how does the big guy feel being encouraged to overeat because he's the big guy? What is it about social expectations and our need to fulfill these ideals? Even though a "big" guy may go to town on a huge meal to impress those around him, what about after that is over? How does he feel with all that junk food in his system? Does he worry about what it is doing to his health and how it'll impact his future? And why is food treated as so harmless when it can actually provide us with the vitality we need each day?

What about the girls we tear down or treat as lesser because of their looks, no matter what category they fall into? Do you know that when you leave your house others are likely going to tear you down in their minds or to their friends for something they find to be funny or out of style?

It even crosses over into food–people are judge-y based on your food choices. It's another area in which we label ourselves or actions by what we choose to eat or what we caved and over did. It wasn't long ago, I was the one thinking about my friend who was a healthy eater, "Man, you are too uptight."

Of course, this was a defense for me as I really wanted to eat like she did, but I *needed* the food I craved, which was junk food. I felt uncomfortable around her for wanting these "bad" foods because she just didn't seem tempted by it at all and really preferred healthy foods. I wanted to feel that way too, but I didn't know how. It seemed almost impossible to me. I instantly felt judged by my food choices when we'd go out to eat together.

Many years later and now I'm on the flip side of the spectrum and am sometimes perceived as being too uptight with food choices. I'm the weird one for making certain choices with my son's food options and not opting to run him through the drive-thru because surely that means, by default, I'm judging *you* for your choice to hit the drive-thru. Yet, all the while, when comparing myself to my fellow health coaches, I still know I have room for improvement in my eating habits. The cycle really gets exhausting.

How do you feel when you eat in front of other people? Do you feel you're being judged? What if you don't order junk food when out with friends or if you order too much junk food? How do you feel? What if you are with someone who eats healthy or is on a diet? Do you instantly feel bad if you aren't doing the same things?

How does this social pressure with food and body image impact you? How does your food on a plate make you feel while eating around others? What do you think about others' food choices or do you even notice?

My point is that thinking foods are bad or good isn't helpful to us either because this translates into, "I am bad or good," and perpetuates stress for feeling guilty over food and repeating the same message of, *"I don't have any discipline or willpower to work hard and I'll never reach my goals."* You feel it is bad if it is unhealthy for you or if it hinders your ability to feel better or reach a goal.

Eating used to be an instinctual act for survival, but now it is a complicated stress inducing process of finding some mythical plan to answer all our problems. This is not healthy nor is it providing any real solutions. At the core of self-care comes the ability to continually love yourself through the good, the bad, and the ugly; to deal with the challenges you face internally and in day-to-day life, and to have the tenacity to chase your dreams and nourish your mind, body, and spirit to support this chase.

So I get it, I do. And of course, everyone's motivations are unique. Not all of you are going to feel the same as me. I don't care what you eat, not because I don't care to help you if you want to do something to make changes for YOU, but because I've been there. I grew up on fast food and loved sugar. Even if you are trying to make changes and fail millions of times, I still don't think less of you because I, too, have been there. And I still have many days where I have bad days and eat too much stuff that makes me feel icky. It happens.

Food shaming is extremely problematic as it often quickly spirals into a toxic relationship of being bad with eating bad food, and then becoming a comfort by self-sabotage with a constant reinforced message of, "I am being or doing bad things so I must be bad which is why I can't ever eat right and lose weight." The underlying message always being one of self-defeat or failure.

We always say we are our own worst critics, which is definitely true. This branches out to impact others though because our own expectations become set for others as well as the judgment cycle continues which *feeds insecurities*. When we feel we are being judged, blame, anger, and excuses come forth because often judgment and shame don't have a way out, or an escape, or an avenue for forgiveness. They feel all-consuming and completely damaging.

The walls come up to protect ourselves and our insecurities from others because if someone else judges something about us, we have to defend it to somehow appease their attack or to win someone over.

The first step in fixing our own insecurities is to no longer feed the cycle by using *other people's flaws to find our strengths*. Likewise, don't tear down someone else's strength and make it a flaw because it makes you uncomfortable.

Don't appreciate your body for what someone else's isn't. Appreciate yourself for every part of who you are, inside and out, flawed and flattering. When you pick apart someone else to make you feel better, you give permission to let other voices in your head continue to pick you apart as well. You don't have to be the best or even be better than someone else to like what you have. You can actually appreciate yourself *and* appreciate others with the exact opposite traits all the same. And both of you can be sexy, happy, beautiful, confident. and content. After all, variety is the spice of life, right?

In my twenties, I used think being confident meant not caring what others think, walking around like you're the best, and boy, I felt so awkward trying to play that game. Of course, as I grew up and worked through a lot of my insecurities, I learned being confident doesn't mean arrogant or lack of insecurities or having some thick skin to not care if others like you or not. It just means knowing yourself— good, bad, and in between.

So you have some flaws or quirks? Don't we all? It's not always about having to fix your insecurities to be better accepted by others. Sometimes it's simply knowing *who you are* and owning it. I'm awkward in social settings, totally awkward and out of my element. I used to try to figure out how to be outgoing to hide the awkwardness, and many times, I really overdid it because I was so uncomfortable and it just compiled the problem by forcing myself to somehow seem *totally cool*.

Confidence is just knowing you and letting the vulnerable, unsure side be shown as much as the confident, cool parts of yourself.

You can always make changes to feel better in your own skin, but it should always be on your terms and with loving care toward yourself, and not because you feel you have to for others or because you are not worthy otherwise. Improve upon it if needed by knowing yourself and then loving yourself more in the ways you need. Improve upon things for your own personal benefit, growth, and learning, and in that process, you will improve your interactions with others around you.

Perfection is a mythical concept of control and a protective shield from the vulnerability of being rejected, feeling insecure, and feeling the risk of putting ourselves out there. If we're perfect then there is nothing to judge or reject or ridicule, unless of course, you're Sandra D.

What then, is perfect anyway? We strive to achieve a certain physical appearance, live up to the manly expectations, or eat perfectly—it's enough to make us go bonkers, and we do!

Another tip—don't take yourself so seriously. This isn't the same as becoming a walking punch line with repeat jokes at your own expense. I mean in the, "I'm human, it happens, going to keep learning and moving on," kind of way. You're a person. You're not perfect, and trying to overcome personal struggles, well, if it were easy we'd never have a good movie or book or motivating song or interesting biography to enjoy.

It also means being able to look past yourself and to see

your world, others in it, and just check out of your own problems for a bit. Now, when you are overwhelmed with a lot of imbalances in primary food deficiencies, this is a huge challenge. I'm not saying it's a simple task, but it's an easy concept to follow.

If you get too bogged down in your own worries, step outside your own box and spend some time doing something out of the ordinary and out of the routine. Don't take yourself OR YOUR PROBLEMS too seriously.

It doesn't matter if you feel bad about your food, your body, your income, your job, your skin color, age, gender, sexual orientation—when you feel insecure about who you are or your way of life, it can be very painful.

By being kind, being loving, and being willing to make improvements, you can embrace positive qualities about yourself and others. By reducing the way in which you judge yourself and others and cease to see others flaws as a means to define your strengths and vice versa, you will have a more relaxed time in being able to continue to grow rather than get stuck in the perceived severity of your own shortcomings.

Recognizing your flaws is only a small step of the entire process. Flaws are seen because of how it is impacting your feelings of self-worth and relationships with others in your life.

Yes, of course, we all want to better ourselves and we all will make mistakes or say something to anger someone else by putting our foot in our mouths. Yes, we all can learn to make changes, and it starts from a place of given acceptance so we have the room to make these mistakes and to grow.

Forgiving ourselves and others for being just as flawed or imperfect as we each are so we can continue to move past it into a place of more patience, kindness, and love.

Stop judging others, and always assume you are seeing the tip of the iceberg only, and as you begin to let go of the anger toward others and the wasted energy you carry by not liking something that doesn't really impact you, the more you will turn this inward. First, you must ask yourself why choices by others makes you so angry and what about yourself is this reflecting? Then you have to figure out how to forgive the other person for their undesired behavior. Remember, it is not your job to fix them, but be present with them. Then, you must turn this inward and forgive yourself as well.

Forgiveness, acceptance, and love is not making excuses, doing the hard work for someone else, or making life easier by doing it all for them. Loving someone through a problem is much bigger than that. It is accepting that struggles are real no matter how misunderstood. It is accepting that I can choose to be whatever role I want to be in your life and in my own. It is accepting the often very frustrating reality of being unable to "fix" someone, no matter how hard you want to.

Conclusion

There's never an ending destination. There is only right now and each day you are given to make choices to engage in your best self, which will include making mistakes because living life without mistakes is boring and, well, not possible. Extreme safety is just as limiting as extreme risk taking. Learn to find the balance to live your life to its fullest potential.

Write out your character—who you were, are, and want to be. Remember, you are much more than your weight, your food, your outer appearance, and inner doubts.

You are this buzzing energy of life and creativity and uniqueness. You all have brownies to share with others and it doesn't matter how small you think your impact will be, because it may be quite significant for someone else.

Give yourself the time, the patience, and the room for growth, which is going to require having room for figuring out all the ways things won't work before they do.

Remember, this is just one piece of a very big puzzle and you now know there are *many* ways in which your happiness can become a priority in your day-to-day life. When you find your stride, even when making mistakes, you will still be living up to your truest potential. In time, you will also find success in your own meaning of the word and as that continues to happen, you can then connect more with yourself, and as you stand tall in your own life, like a strong pillar, you will be able to connect with others and have more to offer others because you have more energy to focus in other areas of need since yours are met. You will be able to recharge your own energy by the happiness, drive, passion, and challenges you take on to better yourself, and in turn, this becomes an ever growing force of life and momentum. It won't stop with you. It'll continue beyond your own needs to impact the lives of others around you.

Now more than ever, we all need to turn inward with more compassion, patience, and opportunities to learn so this can all be turned outward to others, and we can continue to make improvements, grow, and learn.

There's enough brownies to go around, right? So share 'em.

Resources

Katie Mae Nowikow
www.katiemaehc.com
katiemaehc@gmail.com

ME! I want to talk to YOU!! Yes, YOU!!

I will be offering monthly membership groups—you get in a group, you pay your fee, and the magic happens! We dive into the depths of reflective exercises, discuss the nutrition questions you have, and work through your personal hang ups. You will be able to get connected with me and your peers in your group via webinar right from the comfort of your own home for those who are long distance.

You'll hear from me, others in the group, and fellow colleagues with expertise in a variety of areas. You'll learn about cooking (and making it fun), reading ingredients, what do you really want, what's holding you back, and will weight loss really fix *everything?* If you learn it won't fix everything, it'll be less pressure for you to make it happen and to see results because you'll have many things to work for and be excited about!

I'd love to connect with you and support you on your journey. I've done enough writing and talking in my book. Now it's time for YOU to do the talking!

Why a membership? Don't you have some kind of program?

When will I see results?

First of all, I don't want the pressure of making some magic deal work for you to get such and such results in a given amount of time because in doing so, I'd not be walking my own talk. I'd be forsaking you and all the YOU-nique qualities you possess. I want you to have the support as long as it is needed and you can end your membership when it is best for you, be it in three months or three years.

I don't have smoke and mirrors tricks. This book outlines my approach as a self-improvement kind of method, but what will be able to take place in our sessions is getting into the depths of these mindsets, and your evolution of learning will be inclusive of experiences yet to be discovered. I am intention based, I am individual specific, and holistic. And yes, this does work in a group setting in the most beautiful way.

Advertising today thrives on either fear and glamour, and I'm over it. I'm a truthful person. I want you to be open to coaching, learning about yourself, thinking about life, and putting the whole picture together—food, you, and everything in between.

Come work with me!! And if you're LOCAL, you can sign up in person or for webinars as well!

BOOKS & Authors
Michael Pollen – *Food Rules*
Deepak Chopra – *What Are You Really Hungry For?*
Anything by Brené Brown
Life 101 by Peter McWilliams

FLICKS
Fat, Sick, and Nearly Dead
Forks over Knives
The Proposal (Hey, laughter is important!)

Recipes
Clean Eating Magazine – my favorite!!
Katie Mae – for my favorites
Chocolate Covered Katie
Elena's Pantry
Detoxinista